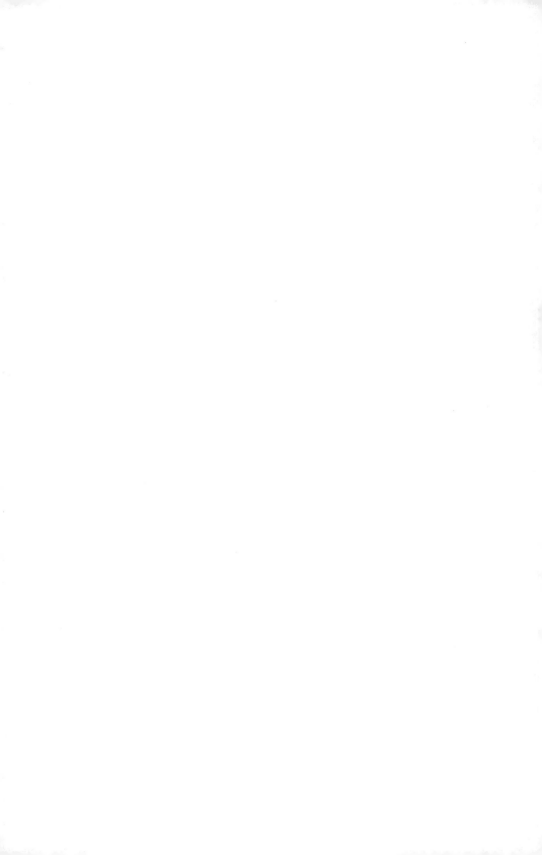

Clinical Magnetoencephalography and Magnetic Source Imaging

Clinical Magneto-encephalography and Magnetic Source Imaging

Andrew C. Papanicolaou

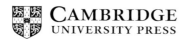

CAMBRIDGE
UNIVERSITY PRESS

CAMBRIDGE UNIVERSITY PRESS

Cambridge, New York, Melbourne, Madrid, Cape Town, Singapore, São Paulo, Delhi

Cambridge University Press
The Edinburgh Building, Cambridge CB2 8RU, UK

Published in the United States of America by Cambridge University Press, New York

www.cambridge.org
Information on this title: www.cambridge.org/9780521873758

First published 2009

Printed in the United Kingdom at the University Press, Cambridge

A catalogue record for this publication is available from the British Library

Library of Congress Cataloguing in Publication data
Papanicolaou, Andrew C.
   Clinical magnetoencephalography and magnetic source imaging / Andrew C. Papanicolaou.
     p. ; cm.
   Includes bibliographical references and index.
   ISBN 978-0-521-87375-8 (hardback)
   1. Magnetoencephalography.   2. Magnetic resonance imaging.   I. Title.
   [DNLM: 1. Magnetoencephalography – methods.   2. Brain Mapping – methods.   3. Evoked
Potentials – physiology.   4. Magnetic Resonance Imaging – methods.   5. Nervous System
Diseases – diagnosis.   WL 141 P213c 2009]
   RC386.6.M36P37   2009
   616.07′548 – dc22   2009014243

ISBN 978-0-521-87375-8 hardback

Contents

Section 3 Evoked magnetic fields

Postscript: Future applications of clinical MEG

Contributors

Section 1

Andrew C. Papanicolaou, Ph.D.
University of Texas Health Science Center at Houston

Richard E. Greenblatt, Ph.D.
Source Signal Imaging, Inc.

Cheryl J. Aine, Ph.D.
University of New Mexico Health Sciences Center

George Zouridakis, Ph.D.
University of Houston

Eduardo Martinez Castillo, Ph.D.
University of Texas Health Science Center at Houston

D. Scott Buchanan, Ph.D.
4-D Neuroimaging, Inc.

Selma Supek, Ph.D.
University of Zagreb

Section 2

Eduardo Martinez Castillo, Ph.D.
University of Texas Health Science Center at Houston

Andrew C. Papanicolaou, Ph.D.
University of Texas Health Science Center at Houston

Hermann Stefan, M.D.
University of Erlangen-Nuremberg

James W. Wheless, M.D.
The University of Tennessee Health Science Center

Hiroshi Otsubo, M.D.
The Hospital for Sick Children, Toronto

Marta Santiuste, M.D., Ph.D.
Centro Medico Teknon

Stefan Rampp, M.D.
University of Erlangen-Nuremberg

Rafal Nowak, Ph.D.
Centro Medico Teknon

Antonio Russi, M.D.
Centro Medico Teknon

Roozbeh Rezaie, Ph.D.
University of Texas Health Science Center at Houston

Mark H. McMannis, Ph.D.
Le Bonheur Children's Hospital, Memphis

Rüdiger Hopfengärtner, M.D.
University of Erlangen-Nuremberg

Andrea Paulini-Ruf, M.D.
University of Erlangen-Nuremberg

Tanja Ehrenfried
University of Zurich

Martin Kaltenhäuser, Ph.D.
University of Erlangen-Nuremberg

Section 3

Panagiotis G. Simos, Ph.D.
University of Crete

Andrew C. Papanicolaou, Ph.D.
University of Texas Health Science Center at Houston

Eduardo Martinez Castillo, Ph.D.
University of Texas Health Science Center at Houston

D. Scott Buchanan, Ph.D.
4-D Neuroimaging, Inc.

Postscript

Richard E. Frye, M.D., Ph.D.
University of Texas Health Science Center at Houston

Roozbeh Rezaie, Ph.D.
University of Texas Health Science Center at Houston

Andrew C. Papanicolaou, Ph.D.
University of Texas Health Science Center at Houston

Fernando Maestú, Ph.D.
Complutense University of Madrid

Alberto Fernandez, Ph.D.
Complutense University of Madrid

Cheryl J. Aine, Ph.D.
University of New Mexico Health Sciences Center

Susan M. Bowyer, Ph.D.
Oakland University-Henry Ford Hospital

Hari Eswaran, Ph.D.
University of Arkansas For Medical Sciences

Ronald T. Wakai, Ph.D.
University of Wisconsin-Madison

Preface

This handbook is the result of the collective effort by a number of members of the recently formed International Society for the Advancement of Clinical Magnetoencephalography (ISACM). The book has two purposes: to articulate the empirical knowledge gained during the last two decades in the diagnostic use of magnetoencephalography (MEG) and magnetic source imaging (MSI), and to serve in the clinical training of new users.

As the knowledge of the clinical uses of MEG/MSI is at present rather limited and in some aspects uncertain, we hope and expect that this small volume will be augmented and some of its contents will be updated in the future. We therefore offer this handbook not as a definite authoritative reference volume, but as a blueprint of work in progress in an ever-expanding area of clinical sciences.

On behalf of all the co-authors I wish to thank Richard Marley and Katie James of Cambridge University Press for their patience and their support in producing this volume. I also wish to thank Drs. Wenbo Zhang and Stephan Moratti for their comments, and 4-D Neuroimaging for their material support. In particular, I wish to recognize here the following people associated with 4-D Neuroimaging: Dr. Kenneth Squires for his substantive comments, Carol Squires for her careful editing of the entire manuscript, and Jennifer Pecina for her help with the illustrations. Finally, I would like to thank Vanessa Fuller who, once again, lent me her unequalled skills in turning heaps of handwritten material into a cohesive text.

Andrew C. Papanicolaou

The method

Contributors

A. C. Papanicolaou

R. E. Greenblatt

C. J. Aine

G. Zouridakis

E. M. Castillo

D. S. Buchanan

S. Supek

1

Basic concepts

Magnetoencephalography (MEG) is the noninvasive method of recording from the head surface the magnetic flux associated with intracranial electrical currents. An MEG recording resembles the familiar electroencephalogram (EEG) and is used in two ways. The first use, similar to that of conventional EEG and evoked potentials (EPs), is for detecting the presence of signs of abnormality in spontaneous brain "activity" (e.g., epileptiform spike-and-wave patterns) or in evoked-response activity (e.g., delayed or low-amplitude somatosensory activity averaged in response to multiple median-nerve stimulations). The second use of MEG recording is for estimating the locations and time courses of sources of either spontaneous or evoked events of interest, a process called magnetic source imaging (MSI). This second use renders MEG a unique supplement to – and, in some cases, a substitute for – EEG and EPs. Although MEG denotes processes involving the recording of signals and their evaluation as they appear on the head surface (sensor space) and MSI refers to processes involving the localization of the sources of those signals and the construction of "maps" or "images" of brain activity and activation, in practice – and even in formal discourse – these two terms (MEG and MSI) are often used interchangeably.

The source of the activities recorded by MEG originates from an electrochemical process called neural signaling. Of the three main processes that occur in the brain, neural signaling is the most basic and direct. The other two processes, metabolism and blood flow, have rates that *depend* on neuronal activity and thus are imaged indirectly through methods such as positron-emission tomography (PET) and functional magnetic resonance imaging (fMRI). The specific events that constitute signaling among neurons include the release of neurotransmitters into synapses and the flow or movement of ions within and outside of cells, i.e., electrical currents.

These electrical currents are associated with magnetic signals that, much like the light reflected from an object, radiate from their point of origin inside

3

the brain to the outer brain surface where, during MEG, they are captured by special sensors (magnetometers or gradiometers). These magnetic signals do not interact causally with the biological events with which they are associated (i.e., the signaling or communication among neurons) and, therefore, do not affect the neuronal-signaling events, any more than light reflected from an object changes the nature of the object. Because MEG/MSI records these causally noninteractive magnetic signals as they naturally occur, without the mediation of any additional form of energy – as is necessary for PET and fMRI, with radiopharmaceuticals, strong static magnetic fields, and radiofrequency pulses – testing is completely noninvasive.

The events of neuronal signaling are continuous, but the rates at which they occur vary from time to time and from one brain region to the next so that each brain structure displays a characteristic baseline activity. Capturing a baseline–activity profile is the most basic step in functional imaging.

Almost as basic is the recording of noticeable spontaneous deviations from the expected baselines in particular areas of the brain – indicative of either hypoactive or hyperactive signaling. These deviations are of two kinds. The first is chronic and constant over time; the second is phasic, appearing intermittently. An example of the former is focal slow-wave activity, where a particular brain area, usually bordering a lesion, is constantly producing low-frequency, high-amplitude signals. One example of the latter type of deviation is the epileptiform spike-and-wave discharge, which will be dealt with extensively in a later part of this book.

In addition to recording baseline activity of the brain and the spontaneous chronic or phasic deviations from baseline, capturing activities that are specific to the execution of particular behavioral or psychological functions – whether simple sensory and motor or "higher" cognitive functions – is of special interest. Such activities are evoked either by environmental events (e.g., sensory stimuli) or by internal processes (e.g., decisions or thoughts). To facilitate discussion, we will refer to all function-specific activities as **activation**.

Moreover, two types of activation can be distinguished: those that are stimulus and motor-act specific, corresponding to simple sensory and motor functions; and those that are task specific, corresponding to higher functions, such as language, that may or may not be occasioned by environmental events.

Describing sources of activity or of activation accurately – or, alternatively, constructing functional images of high fidelity – constitutes a very serious challenge for MEG/MSI. Fidelity depends on both reliability and validity. Determining *reliability* logically comes before determining validity and is usually easier to solve. The question can be stated as follows. Provided we image the same brain circuitry or brain mechanism several times and use the same instruments and procedures, how consistently do we obtain the same image? Clearly, if images of the same mechanism – or maps of the same activation pattern – differ, our method of imaging is not trustworthy. How trustworthy or reliable the particular procedures of MEG/MSI imaging are can be readily ascertained by replication, and in many cases they have been (please see the following chapters).

The question of determining *validity*, on the other hand, is much more difficult to answer. Suppose we intend to capture the pattern of brain activation that corresponds to the function of perception of speech. Does our image represent the pattern specific to that function only, or **also** to, say, the function of attention, or **instead** to the function of memory? Or, how accurately and to what degree of completeness and detail does the image represent the brain-activation pattern we intended to capture?

The first requirement for answering such questions is to know what constitutes the requisite degree of detail. If all we require is an outline of regions of the brain most activated, a rather coarsely grained map of the activation pattern would be satisfactory. However, if we wish to image the entire brain circuitry that mediates some particular function, the picture must have a much greater degree of detail and must show not only which structures are activated but also how much they are activated relative to one another, for what duration, and in what order. The image in this case must possess the greatest possible temporal and spatial resolution.

Spatial resolution may be conceived in two alternative ways. First, the term may be used – and most often is – to refer to the minimum size of an area of brain activation that can be differentiated from adjacent areas of activation, i.e., the minimum size of pixels, two-dimensional (2-D) picture elements, or of voxels, three-dimensional (3-D) volume elements, in which different degrees of activation can be distinguished. Second – and less commonly used – spatial resolution may refer to how many areas (pixels or voxels) of a given size can be simultaneously assigned different degrees of activation, i.e., what is the maximum number of activated areas that can be monitored and differentiated simultaneously. The two definitions of spatial resolution are clearly different; therefore, if the meaning of the term is not explicit, misunderstandings may occur. For example, according to the first definition, one can claim that the method of MEG/MSI, when the single dipole model is used to represent brain sources (see below), may provide images of much higher resolution than those of PET or fMRI. But, according to the second definition, precisely the opposite is true: MEG/MSI, again when utilizing discrete source models (see below), has the poorest spatial resolution among the imaging methods. MEG/MSI cannot detect all areas of the brain that are simultaneously active, especially those most distant from the head surface, a feat that can be accomplished easily with the other functional neuroimaging methods.

The *temporal resolution* of MEG/MSI is very high, in the millisecond (ms) or submillisecond range. The magnetic flux that MEG/MSI records varies continuously over time, is coincident with the rise and evolution of the intracranial currents that produce the flux, and may be sampled in the kilohertz (kHz) range. In contrast, the temporal resolution of PET and fMRI is in the order of minutes or seconds, rendering them incapable of imaging rapidly changing patterns of brain activity or activation like those produced by epileptiform events or normal responses to sensory or language stimuli.

2

The nature and origin of magnetic signals

Signaling among neurons constitutes the most basic form of brain activity and activation imaged today and consists of electrochemical events that take place at synapses and in the axons and dendrites of neurons. Although neurotransmitter release and uptake at synapses are caused by electrical activity (i.e., action potentials), these events do not involve electrical activity directly. Dendritic and axonal currents are produced by the movement or flow of electrically charged particles, or ions, either between "electrical synapses" or within the axons or the dendrites of neurons, resulting in a physical, potentially measurable quantity, namely, an electrical current.

Were we to view directly the variation of the electrical currents at each and every cell or set of cells in the brain, referred to as current sources, and were we to plot these variations as a function of time as they sum on the scalp surface, we would obtain the familiar picture of activity we obtain with multichannel EEG. We would find that the amount of signaling the brain is producing changes from moment to moment in an apparently random manner but within certain limits.

We consider that variation is apparently random because we simply do not know what the purpose of each ripple or surge of activity is or to what end each of the intracranial sources that contribute to the signals is signaling at each point in time. We assume, however, that signaling always serves some purpose, is always the necessary condition of some function that the brain is engaged in. For example, temporal variations in signaling could be associated with external stimulation, initiation of movement, regulation of temperature, thinking, attending, memorizing, or any other activity or combination of activities that may transpire at any given time. The pattern of activity or signaling throughout the brain that corresponds to each of the many functions that is taking place simultaneously is contained in this apparently random variation, and special procedures are necessary to isolate it, extract it, and image it.

At times, however, abnormal deviations in activity take place that clearly exceed the normal range of variation; these deviations do not require any special procedures for their identification, isolation, or extraction.

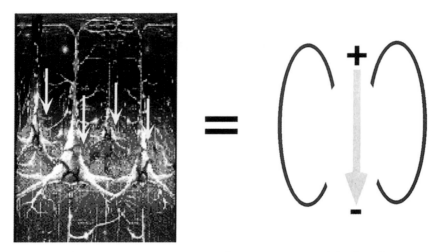

Fig. 2.1. A schematic representation of a set of neurons whose apical dendrites have a parallel orientation. Ion flow within these dendrites renders the set equivalent to a current dipole shown on the right.

Let us then consider what might be the nature of such signs of deviant signaling and how they may be captured in an MEG record. Assume that a large set of cells that typically are not synchronized begin to signal in unison. Their combined electrical currents will create a large deviation, much beyond the typical range. Such a phasic deviation could well be an epileptiform event: a spike-and-wave discharge.

The questions that can be addressed through the use of MEG in such a case are the following. Where is the source of the deviation, is more than one source responsible, what is the pattern of this abnormal activity of the brain? Needless to say, the pattern of activity of the brain itself is hidden from our view. We have no direct access to the source currents themselves; we have only indirect access that is defined by the degree that these currents are associated with other forms of energy that can travel outside the head where they can be captured and recorded. In this case, the two forms that act as echoes or shadows of the actual but hidden source currents are the secondary, or volume, currents and magnetic flux. Volume currents are recorded through the familiar method of EEG; magnetic flux, through MEG.

When cells in a set are activated in unison, they create current that has a particular direction: from the dendrites to the axon terminals. If the cells in the set have an approximately parallel orientation (as is the case with cells forming cortical columns), their combined current can be viewed as a single current dipole, as shown in Fig. 2.1.

Primary currents give rise to volume currents. Volume currents are extracellular and propagate outside the nerve cells throughout the brain volume. They

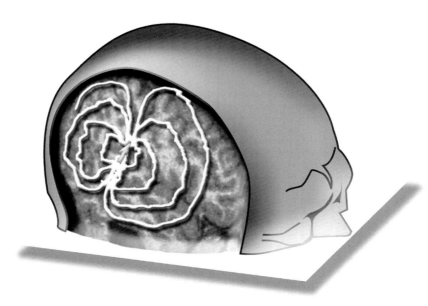

Fig. 2.2. A schematic representation of source (arrow) and volume currents inside the head.

form irregular patterns because they follow lines of least electrical resistance as they spread away from the source and encounter the irregularly arranged layers of various tissues (white matter, gray matter, meninges, cerebrospinal fluid) that offer different degrees of resistance (see Fig. 2.2).

As the volume currents spread, they encounter the much more resistive barrier of the skull bones. There, they are distorted further because the skull is not uniformly resistive, is least resistive in the apertures and most resistive in the thickest regions. As these currents emerge on the head surface, greatly distorted and attenuated, they may be recorded as voltage differences among the electrodes of the conventional EEG method.

The shape of the voltage distribution of these volume currents, recorded by multiple EEG electrodes, imperfectly mirrors the shape of the primary currents from which the distribution arises. This imperfect relation between the surface voltage distribution and the primary, or source, currents makes obtaining functional images of high fidelity technically challenging. Reducing this difficulty is the main contribution of the MEG method. With MEG we aim to capture the surface distribution of the magnetic flux.

As shown in Fig. 2.3, a current is always associated with a magnetic field perpendicular to its direction. The relative direction of the current and the magnetic flux are described by the right-hand rule, which states that, if the direction of the thumb of the right hand represents the direction of the current,

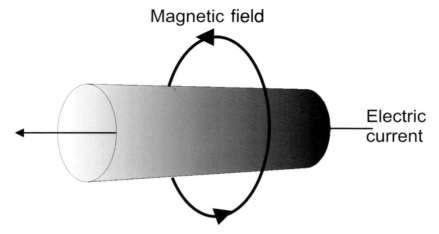

Fig. 2.3. A moving charge (i.e., electric current) induces a magnetic field.

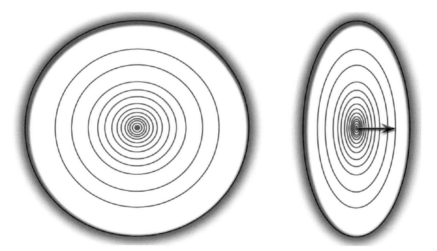

Fig. 2.4. The source current (arrow) and the magnetic flux density lines it produces.

the direction of the curled fingers indicates the direction of the associated flux.

The magnetic flux density – or, equivalently, the magnetic field strength – is proportional to the strength of the source current measured in ampère meters (A m) and dissipates as a function of the square of the distance from the current source, as shown (arrow) in Fig. 2.4 where the source strength is pictorially represented by the density of flux lines (circles).

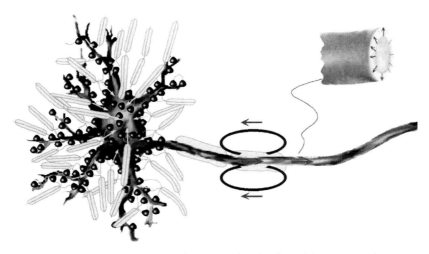

Fig. 2.5. A schematic representation of a neuron showing the axial symmetry of currents moving down its axon.

The property of proportional dissipation of magnetic fields is very important because the constituent flux lines are not distorted as they emerge from the brain source to the head surface. Flux lines could – and often do – result in geometrically regular surface distributions from which we can construct fairly accurate functional images.

The reason flux lines are not distorted as they pass through the various tissue layers is that all biological tissues offer practically zero resistance to them. The magnetic permeability of tissues is practically the same as that of empty space.

Both source and volume currents produce magnetic fields. However, the fields that emerge on the head surface are due mostly to source currents, although volume currents may contribute appreciably. The contribution of volume currents to the magnetic field depends on the shape of the head. Volume currents, unlike source currents, have a high degree of symmetry in the approximately spherical shape of the conductor (i.e., the head) within which they pass; therefore, the magnetic fields they produce tend to be relatively simple. Consequently, the greater the deviation of a particular head from a spherical shape, the greater the contribution of volume currents to the recorded magnetic fields. For more details on this issue, see the report by Hämäläinen and coworkers [1].

Of the three component currents – dendritic, synaptic, and axonal – that constitute source activity, the dendritic current contributes most to the flux that exits the head. Synaptic and axon-terminal currents are not reflected in the surface flux mainly because they are randomly oriented with respect to each other, their associated magnetic fields cancel out, as shown in Fig. 2.5.

Axonal ion flow is not reflected in the surface flux for two reasons: (1) propagation of currents in the axon (action potentials) involves transmembrane currents that, due to their axial symmetry, produce fields that cancel each other out; (2) action potentials are very brief, and chances that a sufficient number of axons would depolarize in synchrony so that they could create a sufficiently strong combined magnetic field to reach the head surface is highly unlikely. In short, the flux captured by MEG is due mostly to synchronized currents in sets of dendrites with parallel or approximately parallel orientation.

3

Recording the magnetic flux

The shape of the recorded flux distribution on the head surface is jointly determined by the characteristics of the flux that emerges from the intracranial sources and the characteristics of the recording instruments. Magnetic flux lines emanating from a source emerge on the head surface as concentric spheres. At the head surface, these flux lines can be detected by special sensors called magnetometers or gradiometers. A magnetometer is a loop of wire which can be placed parallel to the head surface, as shown in Fig. 3.1.

As the flux lines thread through the loop, they create a current by induction in the loop. The strength of the current is proportional to the density of the flux at that point; so that by knowing the value of the induced current, we have a measure of the flux strength at that point. If a sufficient number of magnetometers are placed at regular intervals over the entire head surface, the shape of the entire distribution created by a brain activity source can be determined (see Fig. 3.2).

No matter how great in intensity the intracranial source might be, no matter how great the deviation from baseline activity, the magnetic fields created are extremely small. Typically, the magnetic fields associated with evoked brain activity do not exceed a few hundred femtotesla (fT, or 10^{-15} tesla) in amplitude. Indeed, even the strongest magnetic signals emerging from the brain – namely, those associated with epileptic discharges – are only a few picotesla (pT, or 10^{-12} tesla) in amplitude, which is several orders of magnitude smaller than the earth's steady magnetic field, the fields associated with the surrounding environment (e.g., power lines and traffic), and myogenic activity (e.g., cardiac response), as shown in Fig. 3.3.

In order for such extremely feeble magnetic fields to induce current in the magnetometers, the latter must be superconducting, i.e., they must have practically no resistance. Resistance in wires can be lowered when the wires are cooled to extremely low temperatures. When the temperature of the wires approaches absolute zero, the wires become superconducting. Hence, the magnetometer wires are housed in a thermally insulated drum (a dewar) filled with liquid

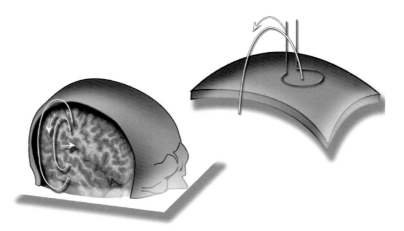

Fig. 3.1. Left: source current (arrow) and associated flux lines. Right: schematic representation of magnetic flux threading through a magnetometer.

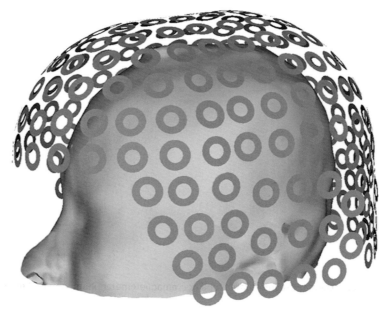

Fig. 3.2. Arrangement of magnetic flux sensors around the head surface.

helium, as shown in Fig. 3.4, which keeps them at a temperature of about 4 K (kelvin). At that temperature, the magnetometers are superconducting.

The induced currents in the magnetometers, being proportional to the extremely low magnetic flux strength, are also extremely weak. To be read

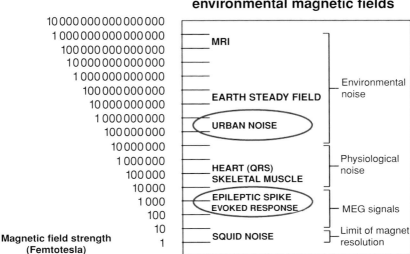

Fig. 3.3. Strengths of biological and environmental magnetic fields.

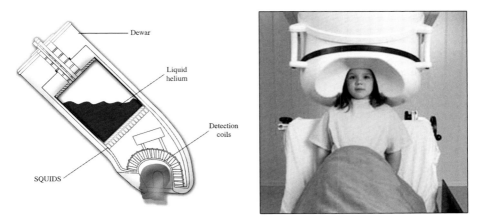

Fig. 3.4. Left: schematic representation of a neuromagnetometer. Right: a typical modern neuromagnetometer system.

and processed, they must be amplified. Conventional amplifiers are not suitable for this task because their intrinsic thermal noise is higher than the currents to be amplified. Thus, alternative types of amplifiers are necessary for this purpose, namely, superconductive quantum interference devices (SQUIDS). These devices convert the feeble induced currents to high-amplitude voltages.

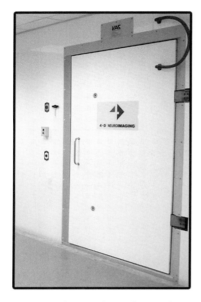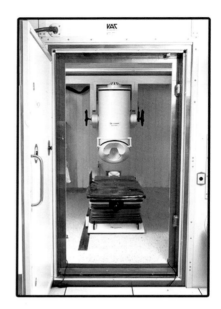

Fig. 3.5. Left: typical installation of a magnetically shielded room with door closed. Right: MSR door open showing magnetometer assembly inside.

The entire assembly – all the magnetometers and their corresponding SQUIDS – is encased in the dewar to be kept at the appropriate low temperature. Dewars come in many shapes and sizes, depending on the number of magnetometers they contain. The one shown in Fig. 3.4 is the latest model currently available, with 248 sensors – either magnetometers or gradiometers (see definition below) – arranged so that they can cover the entire head and record the magnetic flux distribution at all surface points simultaneously.

Given its extreme sensitivity to weak magnetic signals, the magnetometer assembly is housed inside a magnetically shielded room (MSR), designed to attenuate competing magnetic noise from the external environment (see Fig. 3.5).

The MSR is constructed of successive layers of materials with differing magnetic permeability (mu-metal, aluminum, and copper), which act as a shield against both low-frequency – as low as 0.1 hertz (Hz) by $\geq$ 40 decibels (dB) – and high-frequency – up to 1 gigahertz (GHz) at 60 dB – signals. The shape of the flux distribution that is measured results from interactions between the sensor design of the instrument and the density, or strength, of the magnetic field that emerges from the brain. The recording instruments condition, or sample, the actual electromagnetic signals in the following way.

At any point on the head surface the flux that actually emerges from the head has a specific density, or intensity, value. However, only a fraction of that value

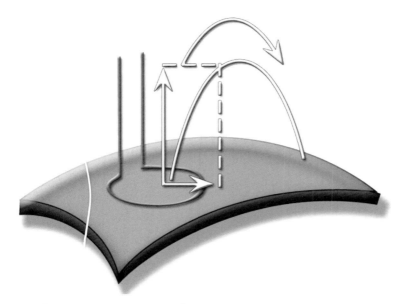

Fig. 3.6. The two component magnetic flux vectors.

will be reflected in the intensity of the induced signal in the magnetometer, namely, the component of the flux that threads through the loop at right angles to the surface of the sensor loop(s) (see Fig. 3.1). Specifically, any flux line can be represented by two vector quantities, one perpendicular to the loop and one parallel to it (see Fig. 3.6).

The induced signal is proportional to the vertical vector only, so that flux lines that are almost perpendicular to the head surface – and, therefore, perpendicular to the sensor loop – induce maximum signal, but those that are almost parallel to the loop induce zero signal. In fact, flux lines are entirely parallel to the head surface (and to the sensor loops) at the point where they are the most dense (strongest), i.e., right over the brain source, as shown in Fig. 3.7.

At position #3, although the total magnetic flux is the most intense, no signal is recorded because the flux lines are parallel to the loop of the magnetometer. At positions #1 and #5, the flux is weak so that minimum signal is recorded. Here, although they are almost perpendicular to the head surface and to the loops, the flux lines are very sparse; the field is weaker because of its greater distance from the source. At positions #2 and #4, where the most flux lines are closest to perpendicular, the greatest signal is recorded in the sensor.

Thus, the shape of the signals that are recorded is not identical to the shape of the magnetic flux distribution that is, in principle, present on the head surface; the shape is different because of the recording instrument. Such distributions, associated with a surge in activity from a brain source (a source that behaves

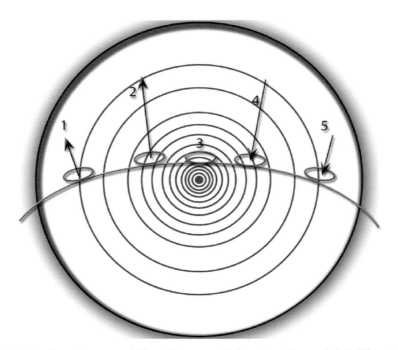

Fig. 3.7. A schematic representation of the magnetic flux strength recorded at different distances from the intracranial source (black dot).

like a current dipole), have a distinctive appearance and are called dipolar distributions.

The dipolar distribution obtained from a set of magnetometers has two modal points called extrema where the recorded signal has the highest magnitude (see Fig. 3.8). One is called the maximum extremum (the point at which the flux exits), and the other, the minimum extremum (where the flux re-enters the head). Around each extremum, the signal diminishes progressively, forming isofield contours. The signal becomes zero at the midpoint between the two extrema and at the points farthest from the source.

The shape of the recorded magnetic flux distribution outside the head surface will have a different appearance when sensors other than magnetometers, i.e., gradiometers, are used to measure the field. Two types of gradiometer sensors are common in current MEG systems.

Gradiometer sensors are used as a means of reducing noise, i.e., the external magnetic activity from sources other than the brain, typically from outside the MSR used for testing. Gradiometers reduce external noise because they are intrinsically spatial filters that preferentially respond to sources of magnetic fields which are close rather than far away. Magnetic fields at any given location

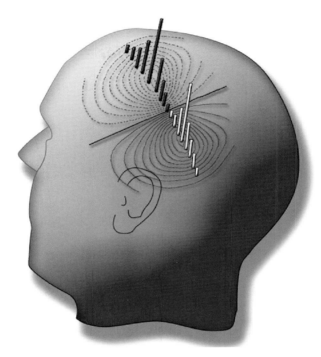

Fig. 3.8. The recorded magnetic field strength (vertical lines) at different points of the isofield map, including the two extrema.

can be thought of as a sum of different field types: a uniform component, a first-gradient component, a second-gradient component, and so on. Magnetometers respond to the total field including the uniform, or zeroth-order, component. Gradiometers of the first order will reject the uniform component; those of the second order will reject uniform and first gradients, etc. All current MEG systems use either magnetometers or gradiometers of the first order. The three types of sensors typically used are shown in Fig. 3.9.

First-order gradiometers reject the uniform component of a magnetic field because of their construction. Their two loops are wound in opposite directions, so that the same flux lines (i.e., a uniform field) threading through them will induce current of the same strength but opposite polarity (+ and −), and their sum will be zero net current. The two loops can, in principle, be located anywhere relative to one another as long as they face in the same direction. In practice, two primary construction techniques, referred to as axial and planar, are used to create gradiometer sensors; both are shown in Fig. 3.9. Axial is so named because the second loop is located along the axis of the first loop; planar, because the second loop is located in the plane of the first loop. Both

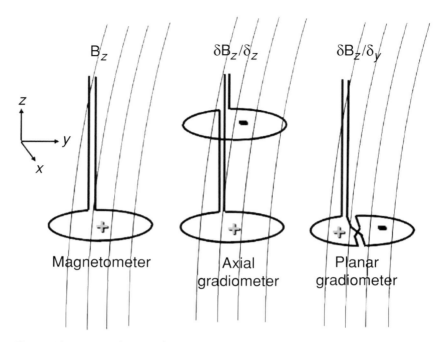

Fig. 3.9. Three types of sensors for MEG systems.

types will provide zero signal for a uniform field, and both will provide a signal proportional to a first-order gradient of the field: a radial gradient in the case of an axial gradiometer, a transverse gradient for a planar. That signal will also be proportional to the baseline (the distance between the two loops) of the gradiometer. The longer the baseline, the larger the signal produced. Longer baselines make better sensors.

Gradiometers reduce external noise because the relative size of the components of a magnetic field changes significantly with the distance of the source of the field from the sensor. For close sources, e.g., those inside the brain, the first-order gradient is between 50% and 90% of the total field. For distant sources outside the MSR, this value drops to well below 1%. Therefore, gradiometer sensors can reduce signals by only 10% to 50%, while reducing noise by over 99%. Using gradiometers is one method for increasing the signal-to-noise ratio (SNR) of measurements.

While magnetometers provide the best signal, gradiometers are better at noise reduction. As a result, a number of MEG systems are being built with first-order gradiometers.

The way gradiometer sensors convert a field to a measured signal is different from what was described above for magnetometers. For axial gradiometers the

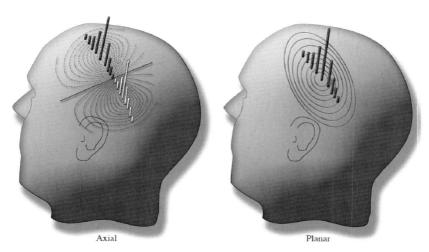

Axial   Planar

Fig. 3.10. Plots of signals measured by axial and planar gradiometers from the same source. Axial gradiometer signal isocontours shown on the left differ little from those produced by magnetometer sensors. Planar gradiometer signal magnitude isocontours are shown on the right for the same source.

change is minimal since the second coil, which cancels distant noise, is far from the head and not greatly affected by the sources of interest inside the head. The resulting measured signals are very similar to those measured by magnetometers. Compare the magnetometer distribution shown in Fig. 3.8 with the axial gradiometer distribution on the left panel of Fig. 3.10.

Planar gradiometers, however, convert magnetic fields to measured signals in a way that is dramatically different from magnetometers. Instead of principally responding to the radial component of the magnetic field, planar gradiometers respond to the change in the radial component as you move across the scalp, which results in the type of isocontours shown on the right side of Fig. 3.10. The maximum response is immediately over the current source because this is where the radial field is changing the fastest. In fact, at the zero line of the radial/axial contour the radial field is changing from positive $(+)$ to negative $(-)$, so the planar gradiometer's two loops, which have a positive $(+)$ and negative $(-)$ response, respectively, would, in fact, add the two signals together: the positive signal times the positive loop plus the negative signal times the negative loop.

The advantage of planar gradiometers resides principally in the ability to manufacture them using standard thin-film techniques developed for the semi-conductor industry. In theory, ease in manufacturing could lead to more precise and less expensive sensors. In practice, the increase in precision is minimal, and because of low production volumes, the cost savings are also minimal. The principal disadvantage of planar gradiometers is that the length of baseline is limited by the geometry of the head. MEG measurement locations, like those of EEG, are arrayed around the head over a finite surface. The maximum baseline that can be achieved with planar gradiometers is between approximately 50% and 75% of the spacing between these measurement locations because the sensors cannot overlap. If the design requires a denser array of measurement locations – generally a desirable option – the baseline must be reduced; this reduces signal size, a generally negative requirement. Planar gradiometers introduce another design trade-off to contend with, since the size of the signal they measure at any given location over the head depends on their orientation. To completely characterize the planar field at a given measurement point, two orthogonal planar sensors are required at each location. Typically, planar gradiometer-based systems are constructed in this way. For spatial displays of the data, such as a contour plot or intensity display, the planar gradient could be plotted as shown in Fig. 3.10. More typically, the fields are converted to their radial equivalent using a model-dependent interpolation routine.

The principal advantage of radial gradiometers is that, since heads have a similar geometry, baselines can be longer, resulting in better amplified signals. The direction of the baseline is away from the head and is not affected by the density of measurement locations required. The disadvantage of radial gradiometers is that, due to their inherent 3-D structure, the coils must be manufactured by hand.

4

Overview of MSI using the single equivalent current dipole (ECD) model as an example

Based on the characteristics of good dipolar distributions obtained with magnetometers and axial gradiometers, we can estimate some of the attributes of the source inside the brain: (1) the source must be below the midpoint between the extrema; (2) the source must be at a depth proportional to the distance between the extrema, i.e., a source close to the surface of the brain produces extrema that are close together, while a deeper source produces extrema that are farther apart; (3) for a given depth, the strength of the source would be reflected in the absolute intensity of the flux recorded; and (4) the orientation of the source is reflected in the relative orientation of the extrema on the head surface.

In general, when a physical phenomenon is regulated by known laws and one knows the causes of the phenomenon, one can predict the phenomenon uniquely. Calculating an effect – or predicting a phenomenon – from a set of known causes or antecedent conditions is called the solution of the "forward problem." The more precise the knowledge of the antecedent conditions, the more accurately their effect can be calculated. With no uncertainty about the validity of the solution, the solution is unique.

The relation of the characteristics of intracranial currents (the cause) to the magnetic distribution that such a source would produce on a particular surface (the effect) is specified by the Biot–Savart Law for a dipole in free space. This law allows us to specify the shape of the recorded distribution that a source in the brain produces on the head surface if we know (1) the strength of the source, (2) its orientation with respect to the head surface, and (3) its precise location in space defined by the three Cartesian coordinates. Of course, we do not have such prior knowledge except for some hints based on the shape of distribution. We therefore hypothesize that the approximate values for the five source parameters (strength, orientation, and location along the x-, y-, and z-axes) that we can estimate from the shape of the recorded distribution are its actual values, and we solve the forward problem. The solution results in a hypothetical distribution. Next, we compare the actual and the hypothetical distributions. If they do not match, we then change, one at a time, each value of the five parameters that define the source, and we repeat the solution and the comparison between the actual and the hypothetical distributions each time. This iterative procedure comes to an end when the actual and the hypothetical distributions match to our satisfaction (i.e., they reach a preset criterion of similarity). At that point, we accept the values that define the hypothetical source as the values of the real source.

The iterative procedure provides a solution to the *inverse problem*. Our intention is to derive from the perfectly known phenomenon, i.e., the effect (the actual flux distribution), the imperfectly known causes of the phenomenon (the five parameters of the source). But the inverse problem, unlike the forward problem, does not have a unique solution. Even if the hypothetical source parameters allowed us to calculate a distribution identical to the actual one, we would still remain uncertain about the validity of the solution because a slightly different combination of values of the five parameters of the source – or a combination of more than one source – can produce the same distribution. In general, perfect knowledge of the effect can only lead to probable knowledge of the cause. In spite of this uncertainty, inherent in the inverse problem, such estimates of brain sources have been quite accurate when certain assumptions are made concerning the source and head model, when constraints are applied to the problem, and when the brain activity is dominated by a small number of sources. Further questions of the validity of MEG/MSI results will be addressed in a subsequent section.

Having accepted the solution of the inverse problem, we are left with a set of five numbers that specify the source of the activity but with no image. We have the strength of the source, its orientation, and its position within a system of coordinates, and the task is to identify the particular brain structure that contains the estimated source. Anticipating this task, before recording the flux distribution, we take the following measures. Three fiducial points are defined on the head surface. Usually they are clear anatomical landmarks, like the two preauricular points and the nasion. These three points define the MEG head-centered coordinate system and the position of the magnetometers relative to it. The line between the preauricular points defines the y-axis of the coordinate system. The line between the nasion and the midpoint of the x-axis, and perpendicular to it, defines the x-axis, and the line perpendicular to the x–y plane, passing through the intersection of the x- and y-axes, defines the z-axis of the coordinate system, as shown in Fig. 4.1.

Thus, the position of the recorded distribution – or the distance of each point of the head surface from the origin of the z-, y-, and z-coordinates – is known, a procedure commonly referred to as *coregistration*. Also, the position and relative orientation of the source is defined with reference to this coordinate system. Often, lipid markers (e.g., vitamin E pills) are attached at these three fiducial points, and a structural MRI is taken, either before or after

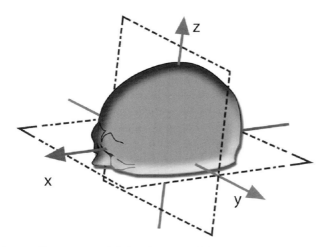

Fig. 4.1. The coordinate system defining the space of the MEG measurements.

the MEG recording session; the positions of the markers are visible on the MRI scans. Some laboratories identify the fiducial points on the reconstructed MRI surface and use additional points (1000 to 4000), digitized from the head surface at the time of the MEG study, to conduct a least-squares fit between the reconstructed head surface from MRI and the digitized fiducial/head-surface points. Ultimately, the relative position of all brain structures with respect to the position of the source of activity is known and makes possible coregistration of the MEG/MSI-derived active source and the structural MRI.

5

The fundamental problems of MSI

The allure and promise of MEG lies in its ability, noninvasively and on a millisecond time scale, to measure events that allow us to make inferences regarding the locations, orientations, time courses, and strengths of the source regions that produced the measured signals. This process has been named variously "source estimation," "source analysis," "source localization," "source imaging," or "bioelectromagnetic inversion." Each term reflects one aspect of MEG. *Source estimation* is an umbrella term that emphasizes both the statistical inference and the inherent uncertainty involved in deriving intracranial sources that give rise to the magnetic activity recorded on the head surface. *Source localization* refers specifically to the problem of determining the spatial location of these brain sources or "generators." *Source analysis* emphasizes the conceptual analyses or the model building involved in using a relatively small number of discrete (typically dipolar) sources. *Source imaging* emphasizes the kinship of MSI to other imaging modalities, such as MRI, but tends to blur some of the uncertainty inherent in the estimation problem. Finally, the term *bioelectromagnetic inversion* emphasizes the reliance of the process on electromagnetic theory.

Regardless of the name used to identify the MSI process, an inherent uncertainty always exists in the estimates obtained. In fact, that there can be no unambiguous characterization of the intracranial generators has been known since the middle of the nineteenth century [2]. This uncertainty is intrinsic to the nature of the process and cannot be removed by inventing clever algorithms or by conducting extremely accurate measurements. The causes of the uncertainty are embedded in the physics of the magnetic field and may be summarized as follows. The head is a conducting volume bounded by a highly resistive skull, and all of the current sources lie inside; whereas, all of the sensors measuring the magnetic field generated by the intracranial currents lie outside. On the time and space scales used in MEG measurements – roughly, sampling events with millisecond accuracy sampled with sensors spaced a few centimeters apart – the Maxwell equations dictate that, if the magnetic field is known on some surface that encloses all relevant current sources – say, the surface of the head – then no additional information is gained from knowing the field on some other surface. In other words, all of the measurements can be simply mapped onto some 2-D surface, which, in practice, is the surface of the head. However, the fact that the head interior is a 3-D volume means that, even in the case of perfect measurement, not enough information on the 2-D surface will exist to uniquely characterize all possible geometrical configurations of sources inside the 3-D head volume, i.e., an infinite number of source arrangements or distributions are possible that will produce identical field patterns on the head surface. This conundrum is the so-called *infinite mixture problem.*

In reality, the problem is even worse due to the existence of "invisible sources." Radial sources in a spherical volume conductor do not produce a magnetic field outside that volume. Theoretically, this rule holds true for the head as well. Therefore, one can add or subtract radial sources at will and the measurement system will remain completely blind to these modifications. This is the *invisible source problem.* However, the main factor compromising the sensitivity of MEG turns out to be source depth, not orientation. Hillebrand and Barnes [3], using MRI-extracted cortical surfaces to construct all possible single source elements, have shown that thin strips of cortex, ∼2 millimeters (mm) wide, at the crests of gyri have poor resolvability. The good news is that these thin strips account for only a relatively small proportion of the cortical area.

The two problems just described – infinite mixture and invisible sources – are inherent in the nature of the physical reality, but a third problem depends on physics and instrumentation. Only a limited number of sensors cover the head surface where the fields are recorded, and these sensors are spaced 2 to 3 centimeters (cm) apart (the details vary from system to system). Because signal quality deteriorates as the sensors become smaller, current technology – and the requirement that measurements should remain noninvasive – limits that number to hundreds of sensors, even though, ideally, their number should be in the thousands or even millions. This problem is referred to as the *instrumentation problem.*

Clearly, not too many options exist for identifying sources that cannot be seen, i.e., the invisible source problem, except to obtain simultaneous MEG and EEG measurements since EEG is sensitive to radial sources. The infinite mixture and instrumentation problems, however, are somewhat different. In these cases, MEG activity can be recorded, but the large number of possible generator configurations prevents an unambiguous determination of the true one.

Procedurally, the MSI process consists of two distinct problems: the "forward" and the "inverse." The *forward problem* consists of postulating a configuration of brain source currents that give rise to the measured electromagnetic fields and calculating the magnetic field that such current distribution would produce on the head surface. The problem is mathematically well posed, i.e., has a unique solution. The *inverse problem* consists of estimating the configuration of brain sources that best account for the recorded magnetic field on the head surface. Mathematically, this problem is ill posed, i.e., does not have a unique solution, because more quantities are unknown than known. Problems of that type are referred to in the mathematical literature as "underdetermined." Nevertheless, inverse-problem theory has developed methods to address these issues (e.g., see Tarantola [4]), so that reasonably good estimates can be – and in fact are – obtained. Typically, such methods employ some simplifying assumptions to reduce the number of unknowns to fewer than the number of knowns. In every case, however, the solution depends on the modeling assumptions chosen. Different methods may give different results, even when applied to the same data. For clinical MEG source estimation, one must therefore rely on protocols – for data acquisition, data processing, and data analysis – that have been shown to produce reliable and reproducible results. This point is so important that it bears repeating.

Over the past several years, a variety of methods have been applied to the MEG source estimation problem. Solution of both the forward and inverse problems requires the specification of two factors: the nature of the conducting medium in which the current sources are embedded (i.e., the head) and the nature of the intracranial sources (e.g., point sources or extended sources). Specification of both of these factors involves the use of models that approximate the shape and properties of the actual human head and the neuronal current sources inside it.

6

Head models

Head models attempt to capture the geometry and distribution of electrical conductivity within actual heads. Knowledge of these detailed conductivity characteristics is necessary for solution of the forward problem because both the primary current (i.e., the current flowing within the active cells) and the secondary or volume currents (i.e., the return currents through the rest of the head that are required by charge conservation) jointly account for the recorded magnetic field. In practice, however, approximations are used, with volume conductors of varying complexity serving as models of the head. The adoption of different geometries and conductivities results in solutions with different inherent errors, and the choice of an appropriate head model involves trade-offs in accuracy, computational efficiency, and ease of use. The following classes of such models, in increasing order of flexibility and realism, have been developed: spherical or spherically symmetrical models, boundary element models (BEMs), finite difference models (FDMs), and finite element models (FEMs). Figure 6.1 summarizes the various head models that have appeared in the literature over the past several years.

Spherical models

Most clinical MEG applications use *sphere* or *multisphere models*, since they can be generated and solved very efficiently and are sufficiently accurate for most clinical purposes. By using external head measurements or structural-imaging data (e.g., MRI), a best-fitting sphere is found that approximates the head (or inner skull) shape. A sphere model assumes that the head can be represented as one – or a set of – concentric spheres, i.e., the head is assumed to be radially symmetrical (see Fig. 6.2). In addition, each compartment or concentric sphere is assumed to be homogeneous (i.e., its conductivity is assumed to be the same at every location within it) and isotropic (i.e., its conductivity at any

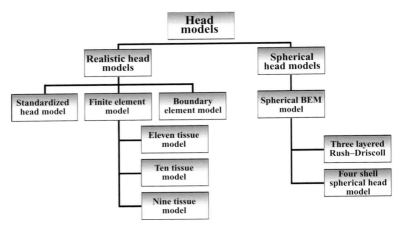

Fig. 6.1. Head models that have appeared in the literature over the past several years.

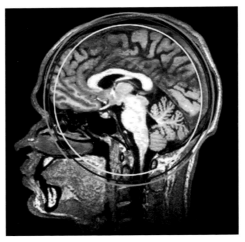

Fig. 6.2. Sphere approximation is widely used for MEG source estimation. This method assumes the head is symmetric, isotropic, and homogeneous. Because it may be represented as a polynomial series, the solution is easy and fast to compute. This method is useful in many MEG applications, especially where the head shape near the source is approximately spherical (e.g., for primary somatosensory cortex) but less accurate for other areas, such as basal temporal structures.

location is assumed to be independent of current direction). The combination of symmetry, homogeneity, and isotropy results in simplified mathematical equations; this, in turn, accounts for the high level of computational efficiency that characterizes these models.

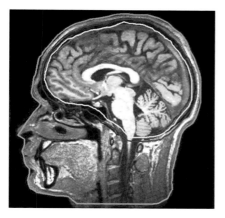 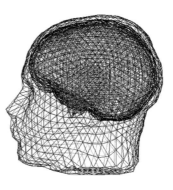

Fig. 6.3. Boundary element models provide a more accurate representation of the true head geometry. They relax the symmetry constraint of the sphere model and assume that each of the compartments is homogeneous and isotropic. The head is modeled as a set of nested surfaces, and the surfaces themselves consist of a set of triangles (right). BEMs are useful where high modeling accuracy is desired in head regions that are not well approximated by the sphere model.

A variant of the spherical head model that is widely used in clinical MEG applications is the model of *local spheres*. Instead of using a single sphere to model the entire head, several spheres of different curvature for the various areas of the skull are employed [5]. The best-fitting-spheres model has accuracy approaching that of the BEM, but is orders of magnitude faster to compute.

Spherical models are most accurate in head regions where the local inner-skull surface curvature is well approximated by a sphere. This is true, for example, for the primary sensory and primary motor cortices, where source localization estimates reach a high degree of accuracy, typically better than 1 cm. Localization accuracy degrades, however, in regions where the skull surface diverges from spherical curvature, as in basal temporal regions, for example. More accurate localizations in those areas require the use of more realistic (BEM or FEM) head models that better describe the actual boundaries between tissues of different conductivity.

Boundary element models

Boundary element models or BEMs (e.g., see Hämäläinen and Sarvas [6]) relax the radial symmetry constraint for the brain required by the sphere models. Thus, these models are able to represent more accurately the head geometry of individual subjects and patients (see Fig. 6.3). BEMs, however, preserve the homogeneity and isotropy requirement imposed by sphere models. Since generation of a BEM requires accurate identification of the boundaries between the various head tissues on a subject's MRI (a process that is more tedious and time-consuming than sphere modeling and must be performed by a skilled operator) but results in an overall insignificant improvement in localization accuracy, BEMs are more commonly used for research purposes than for routine clinical applications.

In the BEM approach, the head is modeled as a set of nested surfaces, and each surface consists of a set of triangular tiles with no overlaps and no gaps covering the entire area. High-resolution MRI data are used to create tiling, or *tessellation*, of the inner skull, the outer skull, and the scalp surfaces. BEMs assume homogeneous and isotropic electrical conductivity for each compartment between any two nested surfaces, as do the single sphere and spherical shell models. However, BEMs are useful for identifying head geometry and tissue conductivity more accurately than the spherical shell models.

BEMs are used to approximate each boundary surface in the head, such as the brain, cerebrospinal fluid, skull, and scalp, using small surface elements; then the surface electric potential in each element is added to approximate the surface potential. In BEMs the volume currents are not assumed to be symmetric, as they are in spherical models. The volume currents do affect the magnetic field measured by MEG on the human head, and by including the volume currents, more accurate estimations of the electric potential and magnetic fields (forward problem) can be calculated, which helps to more precisely localize neural sources (inverse problem).

The anatomical boundaries between two different kinds of tissue also correspond to conductivity boundaries and should be accurately approximated for the BEM approach to be beneficial. For this reason they are typically obtained from an individual's MRI scan. For current reconstruction analyses, computer programs such as Curry, EMSE, and FreeSurfer may be used to obtain the surface geometries. The use of BEM allows for the inclusion of more detailed conductivity information into the model and helps solve the forward problem with greater accuracy. In addition, the border between gray and white matter may also be tessellated, thereby providing a triangular representation of the cortical surface.

Finite element/finite difference models

Finite element models or FEMs, and the related *finite difference models* (FDMs), are used when the highest level of modeling realism is required. FEMs relax not only the spherical symmetry constraint, but also the homogeneity and isotropy constraints (see Fig. 6.4). FEMs allow inclusion of detailed nonhomogeneous and anisotropic conductivity information at every point inside the head (3-D

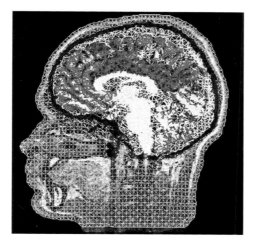

Fig. 6.4. Finite element models represent the head as a set of small volume elements (typically tetrahedra or hexahedra). These small elements permit the model to capture details of head conductivity, such as nonhomogeneity and anisotropy, not available in sphere and boundary element models. Finite element models are of value principally for research.

volume conductor). With FEMs, therefore, cortical dipoles near the white matter or cerebrospinal fluid, where large changes in tissue conductivity would affect the accuracy of the computed electromagnetic fields, can be modeled more accurately [7, 8]. For this reason, FEMs would be of clinical value in patients with significant edema or skull lesions. However, because of the relative difficulty in generating FEMs from anatomical imaging data, these models are rarely, if ever, used for routine clinical MEG analysis.

7

Source models – discrete source models

Both a head model and a source model are required for solving the forward problem (see Chapter 5). The source model specifies the current generator(s) that represents the estimated current source(s) and provides the foundation for obtaining a unique solution. One option is to specify only one – or a small number of – equivalent current dipole(s) (ECDs) to represent the solution. The use of few or individual ECDs for "dipole fitting" characterizes the *discrete source* model. A *distributed source* model, on the other hand, entails using large numbers (typically thousands) of ECDs distributed at known locations on either 2-D or 3-D lattices. The 2-D lattice represents the cortical surface as a *triangular tessellation*, i.e., tiling of the cortex with triangular elements, with ECDs at each of the vertices. These surface ECDs are generally oriented normal (parallel) to the surface. A 3-D lattice is an approximation to the brain volume, i.e., the cortical gray matter, and uses a tetrahedral or hexahedral representation with a set of omnidirectional dipoles at each vertex point. These source models are used in conjunction with minimum-norm and beamformer methods (described in later sections).

Mathematically, the source estimation problem is most commonly solved as a "global error minimization" problem (but see below for an alternative view when using beamformers). Such a problem involves the following. Given a set of measurements, find a set of sources that best accounts for the surface measurements in their entirety, in the sense that the difference between the surface magnetic activity predicted by the postulated sources and the actual (as a solution to the forward problem) recorded magnetic activity on the head surface is minimal. Usually, both the discrete and distributed source models minimize the global error and, therefore, provide *global solutions*.

The second class of solutions, called *local estimators*, does not attempt to account for the entire measured field, but rather attempts to estimate the activity at time points and/or regions of interest independent from one another. These local estimators do not depend on one another, but their summed activity is generally not equal to the measured signal.

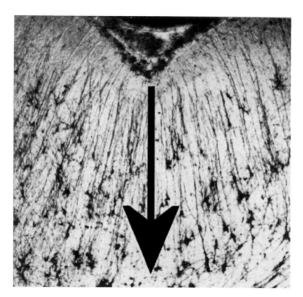

Fig. 7.1. This Golgi-stained section from cat parietal cortex shows cortical pyramidal cells with dendritic fields that are approximately radially oriented with respect to the cortical surface. From a distance, the dendritic currents will appear indistinguishable from an equivalent current dipole (arrow).

Discrete source models (dipole fitting) or local estimator approaches are "overdetermined," (i.e., mathematically well-posed problems) since they have fewer sources (unknowns) than measurements (knowns). Distributed solutions, on the other hand, have more sources than measurements, so they are "underdetermined."

Discrete source models are used most typically in clinical MEG applications; whereas distributed solutions, although widely used in research, have not yet found an accepted clinical application.

Discrete source models

Since cellular current generators are aligned spatially and are synchronized temporally, but the magnetic fields that they generate are measured several centimeters away, considerable conceptual and computational simplification can be obtained by representing a small population of cells (current generators) by a single ECD (see Fig. 7.1) [9]. An ECD is a mathematical abstraction consisting of a paired current source and sink with an infinitesimal separation between them. Typically, current is measured in units of ampères (A); length, in units of meters (m); so the physical units for ECD magnitude are ampère meters (A m). In addition, even the infinitesimal separation between source and sink suffices to give the ECD a direction, so an ECD may be represented formally as a vector with a definite location, orientation, and magnitude. The range for most physiological ECDs is on the order of 10^{-9} to 10^{-7} A m (or 1 to 100 nanoampère meters, nA m).

When the head is modeled as a homogeneous spherical conductor, the magnetic field generated by a dipole oriented radially to the head surface, thus pointing towards (or away from) a recording coil on the head surface, will not produce a magnetic field outside the head. This condition is strictly true only for a perfectly symmetric spherical boundary, but gives a good approximation for the head. Accordingly, MEG signals typically arise from the walls of the cortical sulci, and MEG is largely insensitive to cortical current generators in the gyral crowns. This condition also implies that MEG is insensitive to sources near the center of the head where all directions are approximately radial, though lack of MEG depth sensitivity can be accounted for by other reasons.

The single ECD model

In order to get a mathematical solution to the inverse problem, we must have fewer – or, at most, the same number of – unknowns (source parameters) than knowns (magnetic measurements). One obvious way to attain this requirement is to assume *a priori* that the solution may be modeled by a small number of point sources, or dipoles, whose time-varying activity can account for the measured magnetic field. Historically, this method was the first inverse solution applied to MEG data [10].

The simplest such model attempts to account for the surface magnetic field distribution for a single time point by a single source, a single ECD. Typically, a solution is obtained by systematically moving a dipole through the space of possible solutions, in terms of dipole positions and moments (i.e., directional strength), until the minimum of a cost function is found. The cost function measures the *goodness of fit* between the magnetic field predicted by the dipole location and moment and the actual measured field. Typical cost functions include the percent of variance unexplained (residual variance) or the corresponding chi square statistic. Correlation is another goodness-of-fit measure that considers only the spatial locations independent of their relative power.

Because the magnetic field varies nonlinearly with dipole position and, therefore, an analytical solution is typically not possible, iterative approaches must be used [10, 11]. These approaches often depend on the initial values for the five ECD parameters used in solving the forward problem the first time. The solutions may not necessarily result in the global minimum of the cost function, as they may be trapped in a *local minimum*, (i.e., a minimum within some neighborhood), not the smallest overall value of the function over its entire

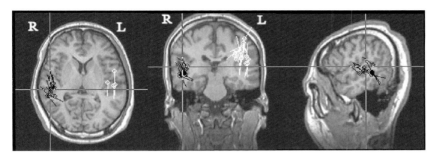

Fig. 7.2. An automated procedure (implemented in EMSE [19]) detects two dipole clusters from 10 minutes of MEG data that included numerous interictal spikes. Data courtesy of K. Kamada M.D., University of Tokyo.

range. The global minimum is highly desirable because it would correspond to the optimum solution, while a local minimum may represent a suboptimal one. Since the solutions depend on the initial values chosen, to overcome this problem, Huang and coworkers [12] developed a "multistart" algorithm (which means that the algorithm runs thousands of times, each time using starting parameters randomly determined from within the head volume) that has been used successfully in clinical research [13–17].

The single ECD model is most appropriate when there is reason to believe that the measured field at a particular time point is generated by a single source. This model has been used with success in the localizations of interictal spike generators (see Fig. 7.2 and Chapter 14), in presurgical location of the early cortical evoked response, and in estimating the location of language-specific cortical regions (see Chapter 24). Perhaps because it is both the simplest and has been in use for the longest time, the single ECD model has proven the most fruitful in terms of providing clinically useful data.

One of the problems encountered in dipole fitting is knowing how many dipoles are the correct number for a fit to account for the field at a particular time point. One solution is to keep adding dipoles until the goodness-of-fit measure shows little or no improvement, or if the percent of variance obtained reaches a criterion level. An alternative is to use an objective measure of signal complexity, such as the number of principal components required to account for a criterion (e.g., 95%) power. The latter method may be supplemented by the use of information theoretic criteria [18].

Multiple ECD models

Two obvious ways to extend the single ECD (per single time point) model are to add more dipoles or to add more time points. Taken together, these additions comprise the *spatiotemporal dipole modeling* approach [11]. As with the single

ECD case, spatiotemporal ECD modeling typically requires a nonlinear iterative solution that is dependent on an initial guess of the values of the ECDs. However, the multistart class of multidipole spatiotemporal modeling randomly selects the thousands of starting parameters from within a head volume [12, 20], from points representing the cortical surface, or from grid points across the head volume, determined from each participant's MRI [21, 22].

A direct search for the location and orientation of multiple sources involves solving a highly complex optimization problem that may lead to erroneous solutions if enough different starting points are not tested. The so-called MUSIC and RAP-MUSIC methods [23] replace the search for multiple sources simultaneously with recursive procedures for identifying each source separately. Classical MUSIC requires the identification of multiple local maxima in a single function, while RAP-MUSIC uses a recursive procedure in which each source is found as the global maximizer of a different cost function.

Reliability of the estimated sources

Once we obtain a dipole fit, we can ask questions about the reliability of the location estimate. Reliability is addressed by estimating dipole confidence intervals (or confidence volumes). One commonly used approach starts by constructing a linear approximation to the cost function (chi square surface) that was found during the iterative fitting procedure. The intuition here is that the fit is a minimum of a cost function and that the uncertainty in the fit depends on the curvature of the cost function [24, 25]. If the cost function is shaped like a very narrow well around the fitted location, i.e., has high curvature, then the confidence interval should be small. If, on the other hand, the cost function is relatively smooth near the fitted location, i.e., has low curvature, then the confidence interval is large, since nearby locations have almost the same chi square value.

In cases where the sensor noise is highly correlated in time, the linear approximation to the cost function may be unreliable. To address this issue, nonparametric approaches, such as the Monte Carlo [26] and bootstrap [27] methods have been developed.

When evaluating dipole confidence-interval results, you must understand that they provide no information about whether or not a single dipole is a good model. These approaches assume that the single dipole (or multiple dipole) model is correct except for possible errors in location.

Although tested for accuracy using simulations and physical phantoms [28–31] and externally validated for accuracy [32–36], the single ECD model has been criticized for the following reasons: (1) the difficulty in accurately localizing more than one – or a few – point current dipole(s) [37]; (2) the problems associated with using point current dipoles to localize extended sources [38];

(3) the number of sources included in the search that must be determined *a priori* [38–42].

Some critics suggest that early activity may be relatively focal, and therefore single or multiple modeling may be appropriate, but this assumption is less justified in higher-level cognitive experiments where activity is believed to be more extended [43]. Some of these criticisms are moot, but one, namely, spatial *undersampling*, is very serious. Undersampling a scalp field distribution gives rise to *spatial aliasing*, i.e., the field distribution shows less variation in space and *appears* to be smoother (lower in frequency) than it actually is because the sparse sensor array cannot capture higher spatial variations (spatial frequencies). This artificially smooth distribution leads to inaccurate source modeling, especially of deeper sources, which would be required for modeling synchronous activation of extended cortical regions.

One problem for multidipole methods not mentioned above is that they provide global distributed solutions, i.e., they attempt to account for the entire measured signal via a relatively small number of ECDs that are necessarily connected. Therefore, the omission of one ECD will generally change the position and/or magnitude of other sources [44]. As shown in the simulations by Supek and Aine [30, 31], if a model underestimates the number of true sources, the time-course information of the sources accounted for in the model can be dramatically compromised as well. Some algorithms, such as the multistart spatiotemporal, or MSST [12, 20], and the calibrated start spatiotemporal, or CSST [21, 22], modeling programs, attempt to overcome this problem by restarting the algorithm thousands of times from different positions along the cortical surface or volume, with the goal of not becoming trapped in the local minima. Another approach for handling this problem is to resort to global optimization methods such as genetic algorithms [45] and simulated annealing [46, 47].

8

Source models – distributed source models

Distributed source models

The single ECD model remains the principal one used for clinical applications. However, a number of other models that are used mostly for basic research may eventually be adopted by the clinical research community and improve the diagnostic utility of the ECD.

In distributed source models, the entire brain or just the cortex is divided into a large number of elements that form the "solution space." Triangular lattices are generally used to represent the cortical surface, while tetrahedral or hexahedral lattices are used to represent the interior of the head, such as the cortical volume. Typical lattice spacings range from 1 mm to 1 cm. Each lattice point may represent a single dipole, or a two-compartment volume (sphere model) or three-compartment volume (realistic model) of dipoles.

Mathematically, these models represent *ill-posed* or *underdetermined* problems, because the number of observation points – the MEG recording sensors – (usually a few hundred) is much less than the number of source coefficients that must be identified (usually several thousand). Thus, when solving the inverse problem (during which a cost function representing the error between estimated and measured fields is minimized) to obtain a useful estimate for the sources, the cost function must be augmented with an additional constraint so that the minimization algorithm can select the "best" current distribution among those capable of explaining the data.

Minimum-norm models

Minimum-norm models [48] constitute a subtype of distributed source models that attempts to account for the measured magnetic field at a single time point by finding the "smallest" distribution of dipoles that can account for the data.

Smallest (or of minimum norm) is a mathematical concept that depends on the choice of a measure or function to minimize.

In the basic case of the *L2 minimum-norm* solution, the mathematical criterion minimizes *the power* (L2-norm) of the dipole distribution that accounts for the data [40, 49–55]. This approach has been employed both in a volumetric grid (lattice models) and with cortical location and orientation constraints, i.e., restricting the current direction perpendicular to the cortical surface [49, 51].

The *L1 minimum-norm* solution selects the source configuration that minimizes the absolute value of the *source strength* [40, 41]. In contrast to the L2-norm constraint, which produces more diffuse, widespread source estimates, the L1-norm approach yields more localized sources that resemble dipolar solutions, at the cost of increased solution instability.

Critics of the minimum-norm approach state that: (1) the results often appear smeared, even for point current dipoles, and at times may become split across lobes producing spurious or ghost sources that lead to imprecise estimated dynamics [38, 56, 57]; (2) the constraints introduced are purely mathematical with no physiological justification [57]; (3) the solution is biased toward superficial source locations and, therefore, depth weightings are often applied [38, 58]; (4) the smeared or broadened effect becomes more pronounced with a decrease in SNR [59]; (5) it is severely underdetermined, thereby requiring the use of regularization methods to restrict the range of possible solutions. Regularization methods (discussed further below) can be viewed as the incorporation of prior information into the estimation problem to reduce small variations in the measured signals that may change the estimated current distribution [40].

Differences noted between L1- and L2-norm methods include the following: (1) an excessive number of reconstruction points can increase the computational burden in calculating the L1-norm estimate since it is a nonlinear problem, unlike L2-norm estimation methods [40]; (2) dipole orientation at each grid point must be known for L1-norm estimates or must be iteratively determined [41]; (3) the spatial resolution of L2-norm estimates is relatively low and tends to provide distributed reconstructions even if the true generators are focal and cross talk between source time courses of nearby grid points can also be high [41]; (4) L1-norms are able to handle outliers in the data better than L2-norms [59, 60]; (5) an L1-norm approach may provide better spatial resolution but results in instability in spatial location and poor smoothness in the time course of the reconstructed sources, i.e., spiky-looking time courses are produced due to activity jumping from one grid point to neighboring grid points.

Regularization methods

Since deeper dipoles require more power to produce a measurable signal at the sensor locations, a simple minimum-norm solution will always favor

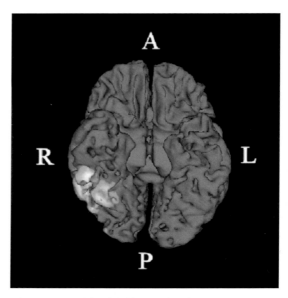

Fig. 8.1. A cortically constrained, lead-field-normalized minimum-norm current estimate was obtained for one interictal spike. The inferior aspect of the cortex is shown. The source estimate is centered on the right middle temporal gyrus and spreads inferiorly.

superficial sources. For this reason, most minimum-norm inverse solvers use *lead-field normalization* (the sensitivity profile of the lead field of a detector to the magnetic field), which removes the bias against deeper sources [61]. As an example, a cortically constrained minimum-norm source estimate for an interictal spike is shown in Fig. 8.1.

The minimum-norm solution typically gives broad spatial estimates, even when the underlying source distribution is quite focal. The spatial estimates are broad because minimum-norm solutions overcome the underdetermination problem by using a linear combination of elementary source distributions whose weighted sum provides the solution. These components are analogous to spatial Fourier components. To assure noise insensitivity, one uses only the lower spatial frequency components in the final estimate, in a process known as *regularization*. Regularization yields stability at the expense of spatial resolution.

The degree of spatial variation or *smoothness* of the source distribution may also be used as a metric for minimization, as spatially smoother sources have smaller norms than solutions that change rapidly in space. This results in the so-called LORETA (low resolution electromagnetic tomography) method [54]. The smoothness measure gives LORETA desirable stability properties, though the solutions tend to be broadly distributed in space.

Several related approaches combine minimum norm with source space–noise normalization, which results in an unbiased estimator for a single dipole location. For instance, *dynamic statistical parametric mapping* or dSPM [43] can be used to determine the statistical significance of the current source estimates relative to the level of noise present in the data. A variation of this approach is sLORETA [62].

The EPIFOCUS algorithm [63, 64], a relative of minimum-norm methods, has been used for EEG source estimation in epilepsy, where there is a single dominant source. In contrast to sLORETA, which is heavily affected by noise, simulation studies have shown that the localization properties of EPIFOCUS are almost the same for clean or noisy data.

Nonlinear distributed source methods (e.g. [40, 65]) have been developed to overcome the low resolution of linear minimum-norm (technically L2 minimum-norm) estimates, but this improvement has been bought at the price of decreased stability. In other words, these methods have a tendency to sometimes estimate a source location that "jumps" away from the correct location in the presence of noise.

Variants of minimum-norm methods, such as magnetic field tomography or MFT [58, 66], minimum current estimates or MCE [40], and minimum-norm estimates or MNE [52], do not generally share the problem noted for multidipole methods. If all sources are not accounted for, the position and/or magnitude of other sources will not change. Spatial filter approaches such as the beamformers also circumvent this problem.

9

Source models – beamformers

In general, a *beamformer* is a spatial filter that combines linearly the output of an array of sensors in order to enhance a signal relative to background noise. In the context of MEG inverse-problem solutions, for each time point, the external field measurements are combined so that the activity of only one current source is maximized, while contributions from all other sources are minimized [44, 67–71]. A beamformer allows signals of interest to pass through each volume-grid node, or cortical surface location, while suppressing noise (unwanted signals) from other locations.

While the current source estimate provided by minimum-norm solutions accounts for the complete magnetic field signal measured, beamformers are designed as filters that are matched to – focused on – a specific target location. The parameters of these spatial filter functions may be selected to optimize certain properties of the current sources, such as location, stability, or resolution. A spatial filter assigns a weight to each sensor reading, and then combines these weights with the measured signal to estimate the source strength at a predetermined target location and orientation. Beamformers may be either adaptive or nonadaptive, depending on whether or not their parameters are based on the statistical properties of the recorded data [44, 67, 70]. Nonadaptive beamformers use a fixed set of weights to combine the signals from the sensors in the array, primarily using only information about the location of the sensors in space and the wave directions of interest. In contrast, adaptive beamforming techniques generally combine this information with properties of the signals actually received by the array, typically to improve rejection of unwanted signals from other directions.

Adaptive beamformers generally have improved resolution compared to their nonadaptive equivalents. The price for improved resolution, however, is paid for by decreased stability and increased sensitivity to modeling error. Care must be taken when choosing the data interval used for parameter adaptation. Synthetic aperture magnetometry or SAM [72] is a nonlinear beamformer approach and is probably the most widely used adaptive beamformer for the analysis of MEG

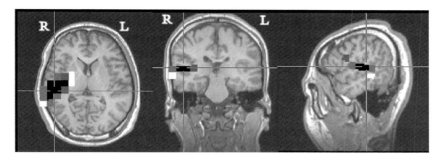

Fig. 9.1. An adaptive normalized beamformer [44] was used to estimate the source current for an interictal spike from the right temporal dipole cluster shown in Fig. 7.2. The beamformer was adapted to 5 seconds of nonspiking data preceding a spike train, which included the spike whose estimate is shown. The beamformer scanned a lattice representing the intracranial volume, which was then projected onto the structural MRI.

data. As an example, an adaptive beamformer source estimate for an interictal spike is shown in Fig. 9.1.

Minimum-norm approaches are considered by some as nonadaptive beamformers, as the filter weights are determined independently from the measurements [44, 73, 74]. In fact, the minimum-norm solution is only dependent on the noise covariance matrix, while the data covariance matrix is effectively constructed with help from prior assumptions about the sources. A weighted L2 minimum-norm estimate, for example, seeks the solution with minimal error and minimal source energy (in a least-squares sense) across an entire grid of a large number of fixed dipoles representing the cortical surface. The weights for the measurements are fixed for a given head model and noise covariance matrix but can also include information about the location of the sources to alleviate the location bias of the unweighted minimum-norm solution, which tends to favor superficial source locations, or to incorporate an fMRI activation map. The Tikhonov regularization, which aims at reducing error magnification, can also be interpreted as decreasing the *a priori* variance of the sources.

In contrast, adaptive beamformers are data dependent. These beamformers find an adaptive solution by minimizing the energy (variance) of the reconstructed source at each location based on the data covariance matrix [75]. They can adaptively select the filter coefficients to reduce the output noise, which is independent of the signal of interest, while passing the desired signal through the filter without attenuation [44, 67, 76].

Similar to the minimum-norm methods, beamformers require no *a priori* assumptions about the number of sources to model. However, unlike minimum-norm approaches, beamformers have better spatial resolution for focal sources, have less cross talk between regions, and can deal effectively with both superficial and deep sources [73, 76] as they show no location bias even in the presence of noise.

The primary limitation of beamformers that is not true for minimum-norm approaches is that beamformers are prone to give erroneous results when signals are generated from sources that are correlated temporally. In the simulations presented by Sekihara and colleagues [77], reconstruction results are clearly affected by two sources with correlation coefficients of 0.6 and 0.8 for a SNR of 4. Small but discernible distortion of the time courses was also evident when the correlation coefficients of two sources were 0.4. Unfortunately, many investigators testing beamformers tend to downplay this aspect by saying that highly correlated brain activity is unlikely. However, one perfect example of highly correlated brain activity involves auditory stimulation and the bilateral generators of the auditory m100 component, whereby bilateral activity is expected within milliseconds when stimuli are presented to a single ear. Brookes and coworkers [78] and Mosher [23] presented dual-source beamformers to deal with these cases. But, perhaps more importantly, cognitive tasks, such as working-memory tasks, tend to synchronize activity across many widespread brain regions for seconds [79]. Hui and Leahy [76] also noted that the current beamformers were not appropriate for directly examining functional connectivity or cortical interactions, given the robust cross talk present in the data. Finally, most simulations testing the adequacy of beamformers, for example, still utilize white noise with high SNR, whereas real spontaneous brain activity is rich with correlated sources, which may or may not be stimulus related. In general, simulations using realistic noise will provide better tests of the various algorithms.

10

Pragmatic features of the clinical use of MEG/MSI

Although clinically useful MEG recordings can be – and have been – obtained with neuromagnetometer systems featuring a few sensors (whether gradiometers or magnetometers) that cover only part of the head surface, whole-head systems are far superior and are, therefore, recommended for all clinical applications. At this point the relative merit of the density of sensors, which varies depending on the model of the neuromagnetometer, has not been established, so there are no pragmatic grounds for recommending particular models featuring more – or fewer – sensors or channels.

The dewar cavity in most current whole-head systems is made to accommodate heads of all sizes, but often, especially when recordings are made of children, the head may assume different positions relative to the sensors. The recommendation in these cases is that the head be kept at the center of the dewar cavity or adjusted such that the area of the brain studied is closest to the corresponding set of sensors to improve the SNR. When, for example, the frontal lobes are of special interest, the dewar should be lowered over the forehead, even if that position increases the distance of the occipital regions from the corresponding sensors.

Whatever the position of choice, the head should be fixed during the recording using soft materials to insure maximum comfort. However, since the head position may shift during a recording session in spite all precautions, and given that such shifts may adversely affect the process of estimation of the brain sources of the recorded signals, head-motion correction procedures can be implemented.

All recordings should be made with the door of the magnetically shielded room (MSR) closed to reduce the amount of environmental noise. To the same effect, before the recording session, all other sources of noise should be, as much as possible, eliminated. These include all magnetic materials that may be part of the subject's attire (e.g., brassière with metallic elements, belt buckles) or grooming (e.g., mascara), and the subject should be demagnetized using any of a number of commercially available devices. Also, care should be taken to minimize all movements on the part of the subject that may result in artifacts due to magnetic materials that cannot be removed – or removed easily – before the recording session, such as dental prostheses or other surgical repair devices (shunts, aneurism clips, etc).

The condition of patients or research subjects and their level of awareness during a recording session should be continuously monitored through suitably placed cameras to ensure the subjects' compliance with the task demands and to monitor their drifting into drowsiness, which is a frequent phenomenon especially in recordings of ongoing activity and of task-specific activation during long tedious tasks. Knowing the state of alertness of the patient is necessary for correctly interpreting the recorded signals, in view of the well-known relation between states of awareness and brain activity profiles.

Although recording sessions of up to a half hour are typical, especially for epilepsy patients, or longer for presurgical mapping of somatosensory and motor cortex (see Chapters 20–21), session duration should be kept to the absolute minimum to minimize noise resulting from muscle fatigue and fidgeting, especially with very young patients.

In most clinical applications, the sources of evoked or of spontaneous abnormal signals ought to be accurately combined with other anatomical information, so special attention should be given to the integration of MEG/MSI and MRI images. Such integration presupposes modeling and estimation of the location of the brain sources of the signals of interest using either manufacturer-provided software, or software from other sources. A variety of so-called third-party software packages, both commercial and "open source," is available. Several examples are listed in the tables below. Table 10.1 lists some of the more widely used open-source packages. Table 10.2 lists the more widely used commercially available software for MEG analysis and source estimation.

Once the intracranial sources are estimated, they must be projected on the subject's structural MRI brain image. For this purpose, a set of fiducial markers, typically vitamin E capsules, are first attached to the patient's head and, then, a 3-D high-resolution MRI is obtained. The actual MRI acquisition parameters may vary from center to center, but an adequate protocol may involve a fast T1-weighted low-angle-shot sequence (TE, 7.0 milliseconds (ms); TR 16.1 ms; flip angle, 30°; slab 168 mm, 112 slices; FOV 250 mm, matrix 256 × 256) covering the entire head.

The resulting high-resolution MRIs, typically in digital imaging and communications in medicine or DICOM format, are transferred to the MEG analysis workstation. At this point, three fiducial markers placed at the two preauricular points and the nasion will serve to coregister MEG data with the structural MRIs. Once this step is completed, a new composite MRI is generated, whereby functional information, i.e., the computed intracranial sources that account for the recorded normal or abnormal activity, is embedded within the structural MRI data.

Table 10.1 *Open-source MEG analysis software is available from several academic sites. Most of these products have been developed in Matlab software, and may be adapted at local sites with user-developed Matlab-compatible code*

Name	URL	Comments
Brainstorm*	neuroimage.usc.edu/brainstorm/	Requires **Matlab**
EEGLab	www.sccn.ucsd.edu/eeglab/	Requires **Matlab**
Fieldtrip	www.ru.nl/fcdonders/fieldtrip/	Requires **Matlab**
FreeSurfer	surfer.nmr.mgh.harvard.edu/	Brain surface reconstruction
MEG Tools	www.megimaging.com/	Requires **Matlab**
MNE*	www.nmr.mgh.harvard.edu/martinos/ userInfo/data/sofMNE.php	Requires **Matlab**
SPM	www.fil.ion.ucl.ac.uk/spm/	Requires **Matlab**
MEGAN* & MRIVIEW	www.lanl.gov/orgs/p/p21/mriview.shtml portal.nbirn.net/gridsphere/gridsphere?cid= login. (not open source)	Uses free Virtual Machine (VM) license from IDL

* Reads data from different MEG whole-head systems

Table 10.2 *Commercial third-party MEG analysis software is available from several vendors. Typically, these commercial packages are not open source, and their development is controlled by the vendor*

Name	URL
ASA	www.ant-neuro.com/products/asa/meg
BESA	www.besa.de/index_home.htm
Curry	www.neuroscan.com/
EMSE	www.sourcesignal.com

Finally, these composite DICOM images are loaded onto a neuronavigation system that may be used in the operating room for stereotactic surgery. In such a system, every physical location in the brain has a unique set of coordinates in the 3-D coordinate system of the composite MRI, and coordinate matching, or coregistration, is accomplished by first fixing the patient's head to a head holder (e.g., Mayfield) and then pointing a hand-held stereotactic wand at each fiducial marker. A set of interactive hardware and software tools allows accurate visualization of the physical points on the composite MRI, as well as matching of contours on the head surface to contours on MRI [80, 81].

A neuronavigation system guides the surgeon to the intracranial target quickly and safely, while coregistration of the functional image with anatomical

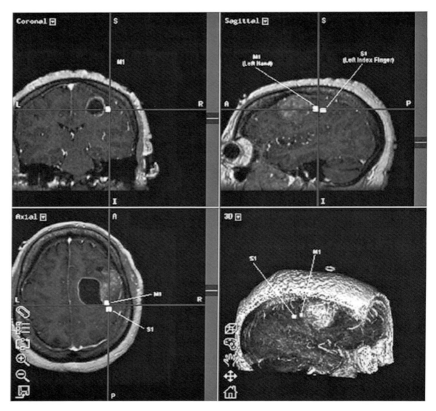

Fig. 10.1. MEG data (equivalent current dipoles or ECDs) representing sources in the primary somatosensory (S1) and primary motor (M1) cortices integrated onto the navigation system (StealthStation® TREON® plus). In this case, ECDs were estimated to visualize their relation to the large right frontal tumor that was to be resected.

image can provide information about cortical areas that need to be removed, e.g., epileptogenic foci, as well as areas of eloquent cortex that must be preserved intact, such as language and somatosensory areas. An example is shown in Fig. 10.1, where the primary somatosensory (S1) and primary motor (M1) cortices are shown along with the lesion.

References

1. Hämäläinen M, Hari R, Ilmoniemi R, Knuutila J, Lounasmaa OV. Magnetoencephalography – theory, instrumentation, and applications to noninvasive studies of the working human brain. *Rev Mod Phys* 1993; **65**(2): 413–497.
2. Helmholtz HLF. Ueber einige Gesetze der Vertheilung elektrischer Ströme in körperlichen Leitern mit Anwendung auf die thierisch-elektrischen Versuche. *Ann Phys Chem* 1867; **89**: 211–233, 354–377.
3. Hillebrand A, and Barnes GR. A quantitative assessment of the sensitivity of whole-head MEG to activity in the adult human cortex. *NeuroImage* 2002; **16**(3 Pt 1): 638–650.
4. Tarantola A. *Inverse Problem Theory and Methods for Model Parameter Estimation.* Philadelphia: SIAM, 2004.
5. Huang MX, Mosher JC, Leahy RM. A sensor-weighted overlapping-sphere head model and exhaustive head model comparison for MEG. *Phys Med Biol* 1999; **44**: 423–440.
6. Hämäläinen M, Sarvas J. Feasibility of the homogeneous head model in the interpretation of neuromagnetic fields. *Phys Med Biol* 1987; **32**: 91–98.
7. Haueisen J, Ramon C, Eiselt M, Brauer H, Nowak H. Influence of tissue resistivities on neuromagnetic fields and electric potentials studied with a finite element model of the head. *IEEE Trans Biomed Eng* 1997; **44**(8): 727–735.
8. Wolters CH, Anwander A, Tricoche X, Lew S, Johnson CR. Influence of local and remote white matter conductivity anisotropy for a thalamic source on EEG/MEG field and return current computation. *Int J Bioelectromagn (IJBEM)* 2005; **1**: 203–206.
9. Brazier MAB. A study of the electrical field at the surface of the head. *Electroencephalogr Clin Neurophysiol* 1949; **2**(Suppl): 38–52.
10. Cuffin, BN. A comparison of moving dipole inverse solutions using EEG's and MEG's. *IEEE Trans Biomed Eng* 1985; **32**: 905–910.
11. Scherg M, von Cramon D. Evoked dipole source potentials of the human auditory cortex. *Electroencephalogr Clin Neurophysiol* 1986; **65**: 344–360.
12. Huang M, Aine CJ, Supek S, Best E, Ranken D, Flynn ER. Multi-start downhill simplex method for spatio-temporal source localization in magnetoencephalography. *Electroencephalogr Clin Neurophysiol* 1998; **108**: 32–44.
13. Huang M, Davis LE, Aine C, *et al.* MEG response to median nerve stimulation correlates with recovery of sensory and motor function after stroke. *Clin Neurophysiol* 2004; **115**(4): 820–833.

14. Aine C, Adair J, Knoefel J, *et al.* Temporal dynamics of age-related differences in auditory incidental verbal learning. *Brain Res Cogn Brain Res* 2005; **24**: 1–18.

15. Kovacevic S, Qualls C, Adair JC, *et al.* Age-related effects on superior temporal gyrus activity during an oddball task. *Neuroreport* 2005; **16**: 1075–1079.

16. Aine CJ, Woodruff CC, Knoefel JE, *et al.* Aging: compensation or maturation? *NeuroImage* 2006; **32**: 1891–1904.

17. Stephen JM, Ranken D, Best E, *et al.* Aging changes and gender differences in response to median nerve stimulation measured with MEG. *Clin Neurophysiol* 2006; **117**: 131–143.

18. Akaike H. A new look at the statistical model identification. *IEEE Trans Automatic Control* 1974; **19**(6): 716–723.

19. Ossadtchi A, Baillet S, Mosher JC, Thyerlei D, Sutherling W, Leahy RM. Automated interictal spike detection and source localization in magnetoencephalography using independent components analysis and spatio-temporal clustering. *Clin Neurophysiol* 2004; **115**: 508–522.

20. Aine C, Huang M, Stephen J, Christner R. Multistart algorithms for MEG empirical data analysis reliably characterize locations and time courses of multiple sources. *NeuroImage* 2000; **12**(2): 159–172.

21. Ranken D, Best E, Schmidt DM, George JS, Wood CC, Huang M. MEG/EEG forward and inverse modeling using MRIVIEW. In: Nowak H, Haueisen J, Geissler F, Huonkou R, eds. *Proceedings of the 13th International Conference on Biomagnetism.* Berlin: Verlag, 2002, 785–787.

22. Ranken DM, Stephen JM, George JS, MUSIC seeded multi-dipole MEG modeling using the Constrained Start Spatio-Temporal modeling procedure. *Neurol Clin Neurophysiol* 2004; **2004**: 80.

23. Mosher JC, Leahy RM. Source localization using recursively applied and projected (RAP) MUSIC. *IEEE Trans Sign Proc* 1999; **47**: 332–340.

24. Sarvas J. Basic mathematical and electromagnetic concepts of the biomagnetic inverse problem. *Phys Med Biol* 1987; **32**: 11–22.

25. Fuchs M, Wagner M, Kastner J. Confidence limits of dipole source reconstruction results. *Clin Neurophysiol* 2004; **115**:1442–1451.

26. Braun C, Kaiser S, Kincses W-E, Elbert T. Confidence interval of single dipole locations based on EEG data. *Brain Topogr* 1997; **10**(1): 31–39.

27. Darvas F, Rautiainen M, Pantazis D, *et al.* Investigations of dipole localization accuracy in MEG using the bootstrap. *NeuroImage* 2005; **25**(2): 355–368.

28. Barth DS, Sutherling W, Broffman J, Beatty J. Magnetic localization of a dipolar current source implanted in a sphere and a human cranium. *Electroencephalogr Clin Neurophysiol* 1986; **63**: 260–273.

29. Achim A, Richer F, Saint-Hilaire JM. Methodological considerations for the evaluation of spatio-temporal source models. *Electroencephalogr Clin Neurophysiol* 1991; **79**: 227–240.

30. Supek S, Aine CJ. Simulation studies of multiple dipole neuromagnetic source localization: model order and limits of source resolution. *IEEE Trans Biomed Eng* 1993; **40**: 529–540.

31. Supek S, Aine C. Spatio-temporal modeling of neuromagnetic data: I. Multisource location vs. timecourse estimation accuracy. *Hum Brain Mapp* 1997; **5**: 139–153.

32. Papanicolaou AC, Simos PG, Breier JI, *et al.* Magnetoencephalographic mapping of the language specific cortex. *J Neurosurg* 1999; **90**(1): 85–93.

33. Castillo EM, Simos PG, Venkataraman V, Breier JI, Wheless JW, Papanicolaou AC. Mapping of expressive language using Magnetic Source Imaging. *Neurocase* 2001; **7**: 419–422.

34. Simos PG, Castillo EM, Fletcher JM, *et al.* Mapping of receptive language cortex in bilinguals using Magnetic Source Imaging. *J Neurosurg* 2001; **95**(1): 76–81.

35. Castillo EM, Simos PG, Wheless JW, *et al.* Integrating sensory and motor mapping in a comprehensive MEG protocol. Clinical validity and replicability. *NeuroImage* 2004; **21**(3): 973–983.

36. Papanicolaou A, Simos PG, Castillo EM, *et al.* Magnetoencephalography: a noninvasive alternative to the Wada procedure. *J Neurosurg* 2004; **100**: 867–876.

37. Liu AK, Belliveau JW, Dale AM. Spatiotemporal imaging of human brain activity using functional MRI constrained magnetoencephalography data: Monte Carlo simulations. *Proc Natl Acad Sci USA* 1998; **95**: 8945–8950.

38. Lin FH, Witzel T, Ahlfors SP, Stufflebeam SM, Belliveau JW, Hämäläinen MS. Assessing and improving the spatial accuracy in MEG source localization by depth-weighted minimum-norm estimates. *NeuroImage* 2006; **31**(1): 160–171.

39. Fuchs M, Wagner M, Kohler T, Wischmann HA. Linear and nonlinear current density reconstructions. *J Clin Neurophysiol* 1999; **16**: 267–295.

40. Uutela K, Hämäläinen M, Somersalo E. Visualization of magnetoencephalographic data using minimum current estimates. *NeuroImage* 1999; **10**: 173–180.

41. Huang MX, Dale AM, Song T, *et al.* Vector-based spatial-temporal minimum L1-norm solution for MEG. *NeuroImage* 2006; **31**(3): 1025–1037.

42. Mattout J, Phillips C, Penny WD, Rugg MD, Friston KJ. MEG source localization under multiple constraints: an extended Bayesian framework. *NeuroImage* 2006; **30**: 753–767.

43. Dale AM, Liu AK, Fischl BR, *et al.* Dynamic statistical parametric mapping: combining fMRI and MEG for high-resolution imaging of cortical activity. *Neuron* 2000; **26**: 55–67.

44. Greenblatt RE, Ossadtchi A, Pflieger ME. Local linear estimators for the bioelectromagnetic inverse problem. *IEEE Trans Sign Proc* 2005; **53**: 3403–3412.

45. Uutela K, Hämäläinen M, Salmelin R. Global optimization in the localization of neuromagnetic sources. *IEEE Trans Biomed Eng* 1998; **45**: 716–723.

46. Haneishi H, Ohyama N, Sekihara K, Honda T. Multiple current dipole estimation using simulated annealing. *IEEE Trans Biomed Eng* 1994; **41**: 1004–1009.

47. Khosla D, Singh M, Don M. Spatio-temporal EEG source localization using simulated annealing. *IEEE Trans Biomed Eng* 1997; **44**: 1075–1091.

48. Hämäläinen MS, Ilmoniemi RJ. Interpreting measured magnetic fields of the brain: estimates of current distributions. Tech. Report; TKK-F-A559. Helsinki Univ., 1984.

49. Crowley CW, Greenblatt RE, Khalil I. Minimum norm estimation of current distributions in realistic geometries. In: Williamson SJ, Hoke M, Stroink G, Kotani M, eds. *Advances in Biomagnetism*. New York: Pleanum Press, 1989, 603–606.

50. Wang JZ, Williamson SJ, Kaufman L. Magnetic source images determined by a lead-field analysis: the unique minimum-norm least-squares estimation. *IEEE Trans Biomed Eng* 1992; **39**: 665–675.

51. Dale AM, Sereno MI. Improved localization of cortical activity by combining EEG and MEG with MRI cortical surface reconstruction: a linear approach. *J Cogn Neurosci* 1993; **5**: 162–176.

52. Hämäläinen MS, Ilmoniemi RJ. Interpreting magnetic fields of the brain: minimum norm estimates. *Med Biol Eng Comput* 1994; **32**: 35–42.

53. Ioannides AA, Fenwick PB, Lumsden J, *et al.* Activation sequence of discrete brain areas during cognitive processes: results from magnetic field tomography. *Electroencephalogr Clin Neurophysiol* 1994; **91**: 399–402.

54. Pascual-Marqui RD, Michel CM, Lehmann D. Low resolution electromagnetic tomography: a new method for localizing electrical activity in the brain. *Int J Psychophysiol* 1994; **18**: 49–65.

55. Grave de Peralta-Menendez R, Gonzalez-Andino SL. A critical analysis of linear inverse solutions to the neuroelectromagnetic inverse problem. *IEEE Trans Biomed Eng* 1998; **45**: 440–448.

56. David O, Garnero L, Cosmelli D, Varela FJ. Estimation of neural dynamics from MEG/EEG cortical current density maps: application to the reconstruction of large-scale cortical synchrony. *IEEE Trans Biomed Eng* 2002; **49**: 975–987.

57. Michel CM, Murray MM, Lantz G, Gonzalez S, Spinelli L, Grave de Peralta R. EEG source imaging. *Clin Neurophysiol* 2004; **115**: 2195–2222.

58. Ioannides AA, Bolton JPR, Clarke CJS. Continous probabilistic solutions to the biomagnetic inverse problem. *Inverse Problems* 1990; **6**: 523–542.

59. Wischmann HA, Fuchs M, Wagner M, Doessel O. Current density imaging: a time series reconstruction implementing a "best fixed distributions" constraint. In: Baumgartner C, Deeke L, Stroink G, Williamson SJ, eds. *Biomagnetism: Fundamental Research and Clinical Applications*. Amsterdam: IOS Press, 1995, 427–432.

60. Ke Q, Kanade T. Robust subspace computation using L1 norm. Technical Report: CMU-CS-03-172. Carnegie Mellon University, 2003.

61. Crowley TA, Haupt CD, Kynor DB. A weighting matrix to remove depth bias in the linear biomagnetic inverse problem with applications to cardiology. In: Aine C, Okada Y, Stroink G, Swithenby S, Wood C, eds. *Biomag 1996: Proceedings of the Tenth International Conference on Biomagnetism*; 1996 Feb 16–21; Santa Fe, NM. New York: Springer-Verlag, 1996, 197–200.

62. Pascual-Marqui RD. Standardized low-resolution brain electromagnetic tomography (sLORETA): technical details. *Methods Find Exp Clin Pharmacol* 2002; **24**(Suppl D): 5–12.

63. Grave de Peralta Menendez R, Gonzalez Andino S, Lantz G, Michel CM, Landis T. Noninvasive localization of electromagnetic epileptic activity: I. Method descriptions and simulations. *Brain Topogr* 2001; **14**(2): 131–137.

64. Lantz G, Grave de Peralta Menendez R, Gonzalez Andino S, Michel CM. Noninvasive localization of electromagnetic epileptic activity: II. Demonstration of sublobar accuracy in patients with simultaneous surface and depth recordings. *Brain Topogr* 2001; **14**(2): 139–147.

65. Wagner M, Köhler T, Fuchs M, Kastner J. An extended source model for current density reconstructions. In: Nenonem J, Ilmoniemi RJ, Katila T, eds. *Biomag 2000: 12th International Conference on Biomagnetism*; 2000 Aug 13–17; Espoo, Finland. Espoo: Helsinki University Tech, 2001, 749–752.

66. Ioannides AA, Singh KD, Hasson R, *et al.* Comparison of single current dipole and magnetic field tomography analyses of the cortical response to auditory stimuli. *Brain Topogr* 1993; **6**: 27–34.

67. Spencer ME, Leahy RM, Mosher JC, Lewis PS. Adaptive filters for monitoring localized brain activity from surface potential time series. *Signals, Systems and Computers, 1992. Conference Record of the Twenty-sixth Asilomar Conference on*; 1992 Oct 26–28, Pacific Grove, CA. 1992; 156–161.

68. Van Veen BD, van Drongelen W, Yuchtman M, Suzuki A. Localization of brain electrical activity via linearly constrained minimum variance spatial filtering. *IEEE Trans Biomed Eng* 1997; **44**: 867–880.

69. Vrba J, Robinson SE. Linearly constrained minimum variance beamformers, synthetic aperture magnetometry, and MUSIC in MEG applications. *Signals, Systems and Computers, 2000. Conference Record of the Thirty-fourth Asilomar Conference on*; 2000 Oct 29–Nov 1; Pacific Grove, CA. 2000; 313–317.

70. Sekihara K, Nagarajan SS, Poeppel D, Marantz A, Miyashita Y. Reconstructing spatiotemporal activities of neural sources using an MEG vector beamformer technique. *IEEE Trans Biomed Eng* 2001; **48**: 760–771.

71. Darvas F, Pantazis D, Kucukaltun-Yildirim E, Leahy RM. Mapping human brain function with MEG and EEG: methods and validation. *NeuroImage* 2004; **23**(Suppl 1): S289–S299.

72. Robinson SE, Vrba J. Functional neuroimaging by Synthetic Aperture Magnetometry (SAM). In: Yoshimoto T, Kotani M, Kariki S, Karibe H, Natasato N, eds. *Recent Advances in Biomagnetism*. Sendai: Tohoku Univ. Press, 1999, 302–305.

73. Sekihara K, Sahani M, Nagarajan SS. Localization bias and spatial resolution of adaptive and non-adaptive spatial filters for MEG source reconstruction. *NeuroImage* 2005; **25**: 1056–1067.

74. Congedo M. Subspace projection filters for real-time brain electromagnetic imaging. *IEEE Trans Biomed Eng* 2006; **53**: 1624–1634.

75. Vrba J, Robinson SE. Signal processing in magnetoencephalography. *Methods* 2001; **25**: 249–271.

76. Hui H, Leahy RM. Linearly constrained MEG beamformers for MVAR modeling of cortical interactions. *3rd IEEE International Symposium on Biomedical Imaging: Macro to Nano*; 2006 April 6–9; Arlington, VA. 2006; 237–240.

77. Sekihara K, Nagarajan SS, Poeppel D, *et al.* Performance of an MEG adaptive-beamformer technique in the presence of correlated neural activities: effects on signal intensity and time-course estimates. *IEEE Trans Biomed Eng* 2002; **49**: 1534–1546.

78. Brookes MJ, Stevenson CM, Barnes GR, *et al.* Beamformer reconstruction of correlated sources using a modified source model. *NeuroImage* 2007; **34**: 1454–1465.

79. Aine CJ, Stephen JM, Christner R, Hudson D, Best E. Task relevance enhances early transient and late slow-wave activity of distributed cortical sources. *J Comput Neurosci* 2003; **15**: 203–221.

80. Rezai AR, Hund M, Kronberg E, *et al.* The interactive use of magnetoencephalog-raphy in stereotactic image-guided neurosurgery. *Neurosurgery* 1996; **39**: 92–102.

81. Ganslandt O, Behari S, Gralla J, Fahlbusch R, Nimsky C. Use of magnetoencephalog-raphy and functional neuronavigation in planning and surgery of brain tumors. *Nervenarzt* 2002; **73**: 155–161.

Spontaneous brain activity

Contributors

E. M. Castillo

A. C. Papanicolaou

H. Stefan

J. W. Wheless

H. Otsubo

M. Santiuste

S. Rampp

R. Nowak

A. Russi

R. Rezaie

M. H. McMannis

R. Hopfengärtner

A. Paulini-Ruf

T. Ehrenfried

M. Kaltenhäuser

11

MEG recordings of spontaneous brain activity – general considerations

The practice standards and guidelines for clinical applications of magnetoen-cephalography were developed by a subcommittee of the International Society for the Advancement of Clinical Magnetoencephalography (ISACM) in 2008. Aspects of these guidelines affecting the recording of spontaneous activity are summarized here.

Head positioning

The procedure for estimating MEG activity sources takes into account the relative distance between the patient's head and the sensors. Therefore, prior to acquiring MEG data, one obtains information about the patient's head position, orientation, and shape by using a 3-D digitizer to register multiple fiducial landmarks (typically the nasion and external meatus of each ear) and points approximating the skull surface. Ideally, the patient is positioned such that the entire head surface is roughly equidistant from the sensors, though in practice positioning can be more flexible. In some cases, especially when a region of interest is known or suspected, such as when a lesion is visible on MRI or lateralized EEG abnormalities are present, standard practice is to adjust the patient's head position to optimize coverage of the previously delimited region of interest. This approach can also be taken for those with larger or smaller head sizes, especially children, to ensure that the region of interest is optimally covered by the sensor array. The patient's head position should be measured before and after each recording block to quantify the degree of movement during acquisition and estimate the quality of the recorded data in the block. For measurements of long duration, particular attention should be paid to the patient's head position to minimize discomfort, and necessary adjustments should be made during breaks between consecutive recording blocks.

Recording time

Typically, MEG recordings of continuous spontaneous activity in patients with epilepsy are conducted in three 10-minute runs (30 minutes). In cases where the patient, such as a child, is unable to maintain a stable head position, performing short recordings of 2 to 4 minutes each, accumulating to 30 minutes of spontaneous data, may be preferable.

Sampling rate

The sampling frequency of the MEG system must be determined in advance such that the signals of interest may be adequately recorded and analyzed. To prevent aliasing, a low-pass filter frequency with a recommended setting of less than one-third of the sampling rate is applied to the data prior to digital conversion. Similarly, a high-pass filter is generally applied to eliminate the presence of low-frequency transients. For most applications, a band-pass filter of 3 to 70 Hz, with a notch at either 50 or 60 Hz (standard European and North American frequencies), can be considered adequate. Since a sampling frequency of up to 1 kHz can be used, the recording medium must have sufficient storage capacity to cope with the amount of continuous data obtained over a typical 30-minute session.

Simultaneous MEG/EEG recordings

When EEG and MEG are recorded simultaneously, as is recommended in clinical cases, using a common reference electrode to record the EEG data is practical and makes montage reconfiguration and secondary processing more convenient. Necessarily, all EEG electrodes, lead wires, and connectors should be constructed of nonmagnetic materials and fixed in place to avoid generating noise due to movement. In addition to monitoring the patient's general condition, simultaneous EEG recordings can be useful for identifying biological contaminants, such as ocular, electromyographic (EMG), and cardiac artifacts, in the data. When ictal MEG is being recorded, simultaneous video monitoring of the patient can be used to compare seizure symptoms with MEG findings. For real-time monitoring, simultaneous display of an adequate number of MEG and analogous EEG channels is recommended.

Recordings during the resting state

Recordings in the resting and waking states are generally performed both with the patient's eyes closed and open. The pattern of the occipital alpha rhythm can be determined easily by asking the patient to open and close his or her eyes and recording each position for 10 seconds. However, spontaneous MEG rhythms should be recorded for a minimum of 20 minutes with the eyes closed and 5 minutes with the eyes open.

Recordings during sleep

As with EEG, spontaneous MEG waveforms change considerably, depending on the internal state of the patient. Therefore, monitoring the condition of the patient from various perspectives is important. For example, in patients with epilepsy, abnormal discharges tend to appear during sleep, so an alternative technique for eliciting epileptiform activity during MEG recordings is sleep induction. Although natural sleep is preferred, sedative-hypnotics can be used, with special care towards patient safety, to obtain a sleep state within the limited time for measurement. Typically, on the night prior to an MEG recording session, sleep time should be limited to about 3 hours to facilitate the onset of a sleep state, though this can be adjusted according to the patient's specific condition.

Elicitation of abnormal activity via hyperventilation

Hyperventilation can be used to elicit abnormal brain activity in certain pathological conditions, such as ischemia and tumors. However, one practical limitation of this approach is that hyperventilation can cause substantial artifact in MEG from head movements, and such movements may be especially problematic when EEG electrodes are also attached to the patient. Some propose that MEG data obtained during the immediate posthyperventilation period may be most relevant. Nevertheless, in the context of epilepsy, hyperventilation is not usually considered a means of inducing epileptiform discharges.

Elicitation of abnormal activity via drugs

If necessary, epileptic discharges can be induced by administering several drugs under the guidance and discretion of the attending physician. The patient and family must be given an adequate explanation of the procedure and its risks, and a written informed consent form must be signed as documentation for the patient's clinical record.

The use of sedation

Sedatives can be used for patients who cannot cooperate with the examination procedure, such as children, patients with consciousness disturbances, and mentally retarded patients. The sedated patient must be continuously monitored either on the video screen or, preferably, by an assistant inside the MSR (magnetically shielded room).

12

Normal spontaneous MEG – frequently encountered artifacts

Muscle (EMG) activity

EMG artifacts appear quite frequently during MEG recordings (see Fig. 12.1). These artifacts are typically associated with contraction of the frontalis and temporalis muscles, most notably during clenching of the jaws. The magnetic activity generated by these muscles is manifest as high-frequency, low-amplitude deflections that can readily be identified by their duration, morphology, and rate of firing. Although more frequent in children, muscle artifacts can occur in a cross section of individuals and can be minimized by giving the patient clear instructions and/or frequent breaks during MEG testing.

Eye blinks

Eye blinks can produce prominent artifacts that are typically identified by their symmetric bipolar distribution over fronto-orbital MEG channels. Saccadic eye movements can cause similar artifacts, although typically of smaller amplitude, in lateral frontal sensors. Eye movements, in general, can be useful for identifying the onset of sleep activity and also can be recorded independently using additional EEG electrodes to measure EMG potentials from muscles around the orbits. Physiologically, magnetic deflections caused by eye blinks are a result of the difference in electrical potential between the cornea and retina; the deflections are large compared to the cortical magnetic fields and are easy to identify in the MEG waveforms (see Fig. 12.2).

Cardiac artifacts

Magnetic artifacts corresponding to the cardiac signal are easy to recognize due to their periodicity and coincidence with the simultaneously recorded

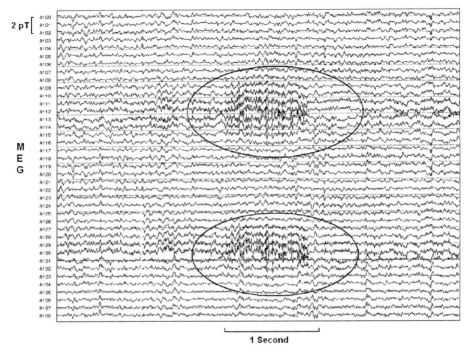

Fig. 12.1. Typical appearance of muscle artifact characterized by low-amplitude/high-frequency focal oscillations affecting channels covering the frontotemporal muscles. Filters: low frequency = 3 Hz; high frequency = 70 Hz. Amplitude: MEG = 2 pT/cm.

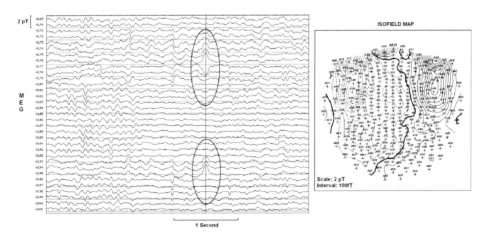

Fig. 12.2. The artifact produced by eye movements is typically characterized by a bilateral bipolar deflection affecting channels in the fronto-orbital regions. Right: isofield map showing the topography of a blink artifact (typically, gradients with higher amplitude bilaterally over the frontal channels). Filter: low frequency = 3 Hz; high frequency = 70 Hz. Amplitude: MEG = 2 pT/cm.

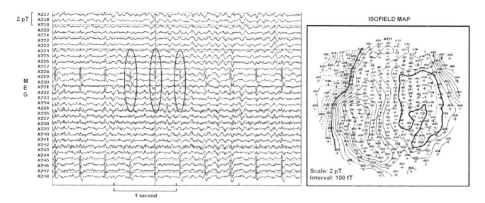

Fig. 12.3. Continuous recording in a 9-year-old patient showing some of the MEG sensors where the rhythmic spike with large amplitude, corresponding to the cardiac artifact, is evident. Right: isofield map showing the topography of a cardiac artifact (typically, gradients with higher amplitude over the left hemisphere). Filter: low frequency = 3 Hz; high frequency = 70 Hz. Amplitude: MEG = 2 pT/cm.

electrocardiography (ECG) channel. Specifically, a cardiac artifact is apparent as an MEG "sharp wave" synchronized with each QRS complex of the ECG trace. The topography of this waveform is extremely variable, but a stable pattern can usually be seen as higher magnetic gradients over the sensors in the left hemisphere (see Fig. 12.3). While individual variations exist, infants and young adults typically exhibit larger MEG cardiac artifacts than older adults.

Respiratory artifacts

Respiratory artifacts can be identified as slow, rhythmic activity, synchronous with the pace of respiration. This artifact can also be enhanced by the presence of ferromagnetic materials in the patient's body, especially in the vicinity of the chest. Although not necessary for routine MEG recordings, several commercially available devices can be coupled to an external channel of most MEG systems to monitor respiratory activity. In most cases, however, respiratory artifacts can be removed easily using high-pass filters, typically in the range of 2 to 3 Hz.

Artifacts from ferromagnetic dental implants

Dental implants are one of the most common sources of nonbiological artifact affecting the integrity of MEG recordings. These magnetic deflections

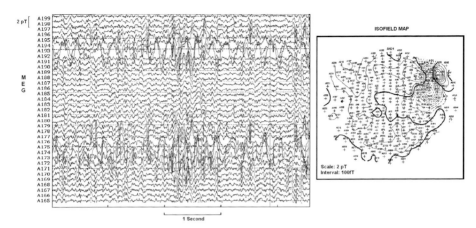

Fig. 12.4. High-amplitude artifact affecting anterior channels bilaterally in a patient with a silver dental crown. Right: The map of isomagnetic fields shows the preponderance of the magnetic artifact affecting the right anterior sensors (corresponding to the side with the dental work). Filter: low frequency = 3 Hz; high frequency = 70 Hz. Amplitude: MEG = 2 pT/cm.

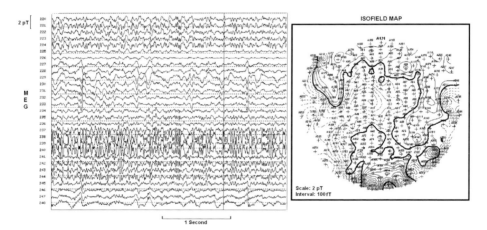

Fig. 12.5. Focal artifact affecting posterior MEG sensors produced by magnetized EEG electrodes. Right: The isofield map shows the preponderance of the magnetic artifact affecting the posterior sensors (where EEG wires are wrapped to exit the MEG sensor). Filter: low frequency = 3 Hz; high frequency = 70 Hz. Amplitude: MEG = 2 pT/cm.

are invariably produced by ferromagnetic materials in crowns, bridges, retainers, and other oral implants. The topographic distribution of this artifact tends to be anterior, producing strong magnetic gradients in temporofrontal sensors (see Fig. 12.4).

Artifacts from magnetized EEG electrodes

Morphologically, an artifact associated with magnetized electrodes is manifest as high-frequency noise across the scalp surface. An example of the topography of this artifact can be seen in Fig. 12.5 where a predominance of magnetic noise is present over the posterior MEG sensors. To minimize this artifact, one should degauss the patient prior to acquiring MEG data, especially if EEG electrodes have been attached for simultaneous EEG/MEG recordings. In addition, one must adequately ground the EEG to prevent contamination by 50 or 60 Hz alternating current (AC) artifact.

Environmental artifacts

The MSR reduces the effects of environmental noise on MEG recordings considerably but not completely. Elevators, automobiles, and electronic devices in proximity to the MSR can generate artifacts, typically in the low-frequency bands. In particular, the artifact produced by respirators varies widely in morphology and frequency; monitoring the ventilator rate in a separate channel helps identify the respirator artifact. Furthermore, interference of high-frequency noise emanating from radio, television, and hospital paging systems can also affect MEG recordings.

13

Spontaneous MEG morphology

This section addresses some of the most frequent normal waveforms that can be identified in the MEG tracing, including vertex waves, the K-complex, positive occipital sharp transients of sleep, sleep spindles, mu rhythm, sharp waves, and delta waves.

Morphology of normal MEG waveforms

These patterns can be recognized primarily by their morphology and topography and secondarily by their frequency. Furthermore, the degree to which these waves can be categorized as normal or abnormal depends on several factors.

Vertex waves

Vertex waves (V-waves) are sharp waves that occur during stage II sleep. Though typically bilateral with maximum amplitude over the vertex, V-waves can occasionally appear lateralized in MEG isofield contour maps. Often, V-waves occur after sleep disturbances (e.g., brief sounds) and may arise during brief semiarousals. V-waves are easy to recognize in MEG/EEG tracings, as seen in Fig. 13.1.

K-complex

The K-complex, like the V-wave, shows maximum amplitude at the vertex and generally consists of activity in the delta frequency range. Occasionally, the K-complex displays large amplitude when coincident with spindles during stage II sleep. The MEG topography of the K-complex is variable but tends to exhibit higher amplitude bilaterally in frontal regions. The K-complex can readily be identified each time a patient is partially aroused from sleep.

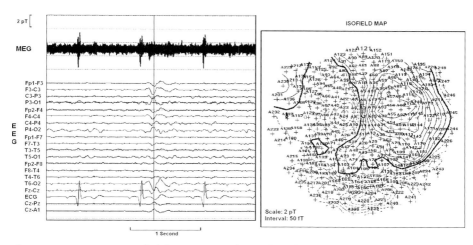

Fig. 13.1. Vertex wave recorded during stage II sleep. Filters: low frequency = 3 Hz; high frequency = 70 Hz. Amplitudes: MEG = 2 pT/cm; EEG = 50 μV (microvolts)/cm.

Lambda waves and positive occipital sharp transients of sleep (POSTS)

Lambda waves and POSTS are similar variants in morphology, with both exhibiting triangular wave shapes, and in topography, with both distributing prominently in posterior regions. Whereas lambda waves occur when patients are awake, POSTS are associated with sleep and are believed to be most evident in stage II, though they can occur in stage I. Both lambda waves and POSTS can exhibit a bilateral posterior topography in MEG recordings, though large differences in amplitude between the hemispheres make distinguishing them from focal abnormalities (e.g., sharp waves) difficult.

Sleep spindles

Spindles are groups of waves that occur during various stages of sleep but are especially prominent during stage II. Sleep spindles are much easier to identify in EEG recordings than in MEG and typically appear as bursts of rhythmic activity at 11 to 15 Hz with variable duration and amplitude (an initial increase in amplitude followed by a slow decrease). Generally, spindles distribute widely but exhibit the highest amplitude over the central areas (see Fig. 13.2). The appearance of these waveforms often resembles a spindle.

Mu waves

Mu waves share some features with alpha waves, ranging from 7 to 11 Hz in frequency, and can be distinguished morphologically by their arch-like shape

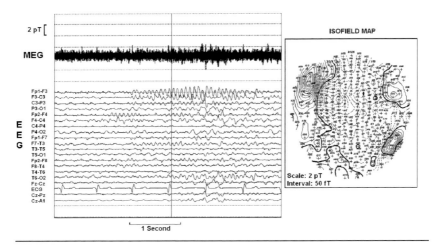

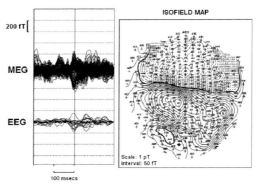

Fig. 13.2. Top: sleep spindles in stage II sleep. Filters: low frequency = 3 Hz; high frequency = 70 Hz. Amplitudes: MEG = 2 pT/cm; EEG = 50 uV/cm. Bottom: amplified detail of individual sleep spindle. Amplitudes: MEG = 200 fT/cm; EEG = 10 µV/cm.

(rounded in one direction with a sharp side in the other direction) and topographically by their distribution over centroparietal channels. Unlike alpha waves, mu waves are unchanged by eye opening but are attenuated by movement or muscle contraction of the extremities.

Benign epileptic transients of sleep (BETS)

Benign epileptic transients of sleep are sharp waves that generally occur in one or both hemispheres, often asynchronously, especially in the temporal and frontal regions. BETS are rare in children, more frequent in adults and elderly

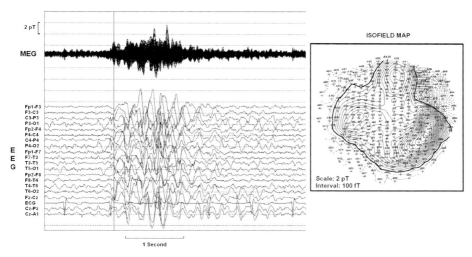

Fig. 13.3. Hypnagogic hypersynchrony in a 7-year-old patient during stage I sleep. Filters: low frequency = 3 Hz; high frequency = 70 Hz. Amplitudes: MEG = 2 pT/cm; EEG = 50 μV/cm.

individuals. Although they can occur in epileptic patients, BETS often are seen in individuals without epilepsy and can be regarded as a probable normal variant.

Hypnagogic hypersynchrony

Hypnagogic hypersynchrony describes MEG/EEG recordings of high-amplitude paroxysmal bursts in the range of 3 to 5 Hz, typically occurring during stage I sleep or drowsiness. While EEG recordings tend to show maximum voltage in precentral areas, MEG does not show a fixed topography for these bursts in activity (see Fig. 13.3).

Frequency bands of normal spontaneous MEG

Frequency is an important feature used to define normal and abnormal EEG/MEG rhythms. Generally, most activity exhibiting frequencies of 7.5 Hz and higher is considered normal in EEG/MEG tracings of awake adults, while activity below 7 Hz is often classified as abnormal. The same slow activity (≤7 Hz) is considered normal when seen in children or in adults during sleep. EEG/MEG waveforms that are an appropriate frequency for a given age and state of alertness are considered abnormal when they occur at an inappropriate scalp location or demonstrate irregularities in rhythmicity or amplitude.

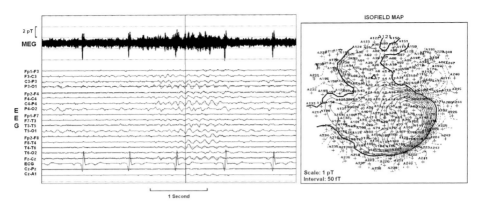

Fig. 13.4. Typical alpha rhythm at 8 Hz with predominant amplitude over the posterior regions. Filters: low frequency = 3 Hz; high frequency = 70 Hz. Amplitudes: MEG = 1 pT/cm; EEG = 50 μV/cm.

Furthermore, certain *patterns* are age dependent, normal at specific ages or states (alertness versus sleep). Although the human brain produces activity in a large range of frequencies (0.5 to 500 Hz), the most clinically relevant frequency bands are alpha (8 to 13 Hz), beta (> 13 Hz), theta (4 to 8 Hz) and delta (1 to 4 Hz). This section will describe these frequency bands.

Alpha waves

Alpha waves were the first electroencephalographic rhythm described by Berger in the late 1920s [1], and though evident in all age groups, these waves are most common in adults. Alpha activity in adults ranges from 9 to 10.5 Hz and is prominent in the posterior regions. Eye opening usually results in attenuation of the alpha rhythm, but mental effort or focal attention can also modulate this activity. Alpha waves occur rhythmically in both hemispheres but are often slightly higher in amplitude unilaterally. Moreover, the maximum amplitude of alpha waves over posterior MEG sensors extends over the temporal sensors in some individuals (see Fig. 13.4).

Beta waves

Beta waves are observed in all age groups. Typically, they have reduced amplitude and are more symmetric and anterior in EEG, though not necessarily in MEG. Furthermore, barbiturates and benzodiazepines augment the presence of beta waves, which is particularly important to remember during recordings while the patient is sedated (see Fig. 13.5).

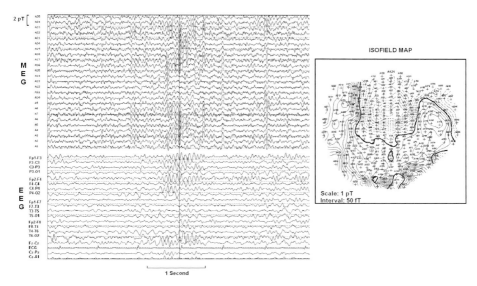

Fig. 13.5. Beta activity (17 Hz) consisting of a burst of waves with maximum amplitude over the left anterior sensors (in agreement with the EEG topography). Filters: low frequency = 3 Hz; high frequency = 70 Hz. Amplitudes: MEG = 2 pT/cm; EEG = 50 μV/cm.

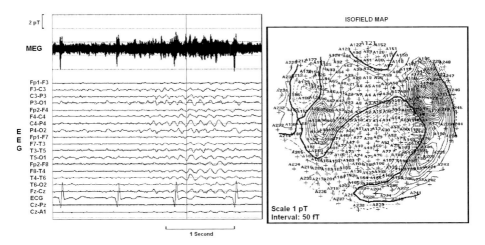

Fig. 13.6. Theta activity (6 to 7 Hz) with predominant amplitude over the right hemisphere. Filters: low frequency = 3 Hz; high frequency = 70 Hz. Amplitudes: MEG = 2 pT/cm; EEG = 50 μV/cm.

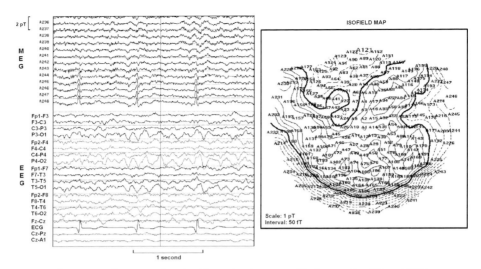

Fig. 13.7. Delta waves (4 Hz) with predominant amplitude over the EEG and MEG recordings over the posterior region. Right: isofield maps showing the predominantly posterior topography of the delta activity. Filters: low frequency = 1 Hz; high frequency = 70 Hz. Amplitudes: MEG = 2 pT/cm; EEG = 50 μV/cm.

Theta waves

Theta waves and delta waves are collectively known as slow waves (1 to 8 Hz). Theta activity (4 to 8 Hz) is a normal accompaniment of drowsiness and sleep at any age and is considered abnormal only when the activity occurs in excess with a focal topography (see Fig. 13.6).

Delta waves

Delta waves have a frequency of 4 Hz or less and appear as normal variants during deep sleep in adults, infants, and children (see Fig. 13.7).

14

Abnormal spontaneous MEG

This section will focus on the abnormal waveforms and patterns seen on MEG tracings as a result of structural lesions, epilepsy, or various encephalopathies.

Abnormal slow waves

Abnormal slow waves, especially focal delta waves, are considered atypical if present in the MEG record of awake adults. Their presence can be characterized using MEG and is often associated with focal structural lesions (e.g., tumors, stroke, vascular malformations), focal epilepsy, or diffuse encephalopathies (e.g., dementias, traumatic brain injury). Figure 14.1 shows the topographic correspondences between a regional increment in delta power (1 to 5 Hz) and the presence of unilateral stroke.

Spikes, sharp waves, and polyspikes

Spikes, sharp waves, and polyspikes are abnormal waveforms observed most frequently in the context of epilepsy evaluation. The topography and morphology of these epileptiform discharges varies and depends on the seizure type, epileptic syndrome, localization of the epileptogenic zone, age at seizure onset, and methodology of the recording.

Abnormal wave patterns

The observed MEG/EEG abnormalities in patients with seizures have specific or nonspecific patterns. Specific patterns are epileptiform discharges, including spikes, spike-and-wave complexes, and sharp waves. Nonspecific patterns, including generalized and focal slowing and amplitude asymmetries, indicate

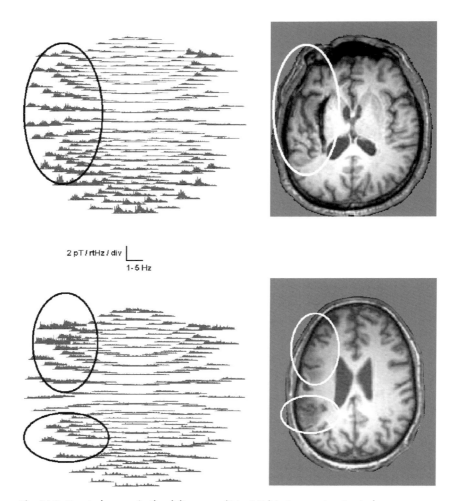

Fig. 14.1. Spectral power in the delta range (1 to 4 Hz) in two postacute stroke patients (4 weeks following the ictus) showing the topographic correspondence between the structural damage (right) and the increment of power in the topographic maps (left). Filters: low frequency = 1 Hz; high frequency = 70 Hz. Amplitude: MEG = 2 pT/√Hz/div.

the presence of a diffuse or focal pathology but are not specific to epilepsy. In partial epilepsies, focal epileptiform activity is distinguished from normal background activity and artifacts by certain characteristics of spikes and sharp waves; namely, spikes have a characteristic duration of 20 to 70 ms and sharp waves are longer, lasting from 70 to 200 ms. These events interrupt the background MEG

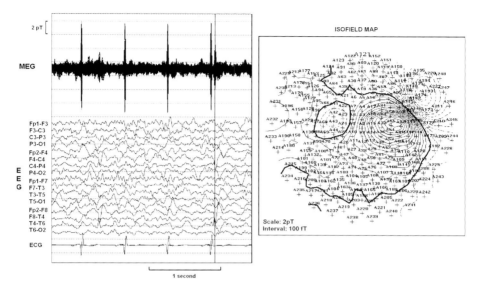

Fig. 14.2. Spike-and-wave complex showing a right frontocentral distribution in the MEG sensors at onset in agreement with the EEG topography. Note the rhythmicity and large amplitude of the cardiac responses in the MEG tracing. Filters: low frequency = 3 Hz; high frequency = 70 Hz. Amplitudes: MEG = 1 pT/cm; EEG = 50 μV/cm.

activity, and the discharge is distinguished by a strong gradient in a subset of MEG sensors (see Fig. 14.2).

Definition of MEG spikes and patterns

The definition of an EEG spike is based on its amplitude, duration, sharpness, and emergence from background [2]. However, spikes in MEG have not yet been formally defined. In practice spikes are identified in MEG recordings by using EEG as a guide, or by looking at EEG and MEG together and deciding on some "general" aspect of transients, or even by directly applying EEG spike criteria [3]. Results from other studies showed that interictal epileptiform spikes recorded in EEG and MEG share some properties but differ in other characteristics, such as duration, sharpness, and shape [4]. Overall, however, identification of spikes by observers with EEG experience leads to reproducible and clinically valid results in MEG [3, 5].

On the other hand, previous studies found differences between MEG and scalp EEG spikes with respect to several morphologic characteristics, such as duration, sharpness, and shape [4]. A 2008 study by Nowak and coworkers [6],

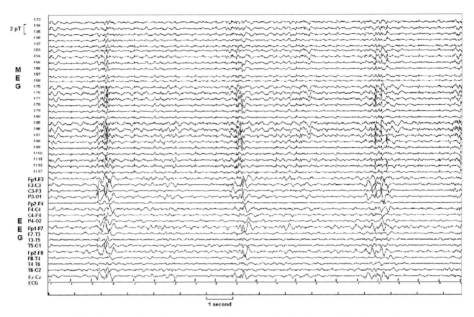

Fig. 14.3. Frequent bursts of spike-and-wave and polyspike activity. Filters: low frequency = 3 Hz; high frequency = 70 Hz. Amplitudes: MEG = 2 pT/cm; EEG = 50 μV/cm.

presented in part at the 16th International Conference on Biomagnetism, provided a descriptive analysis of MEG spikes recorded simultaneously by depth electrodes. Future studies integrating a panel of MEG experts from different institutions and involving a large number of patients should eventually create a spike database and define the attributes of MEG spikes.

The term "polyspike" is used when several spikes comprise a single waveform (see Figs. 14.3 and 14.4). To maximize the chances of capturing these interictal patterns, investigators usually deprive patients of sleep before MEG recordings (see Chapter 11). Hyperventilation, which also can induce abnormal spike activity, is not typically recommended due to the adverse effect of head movement during MEG recording.

MEG and epilepsy

The application of MEG to generalized epilepsy is controversial and should be approached with caution since localization of generalized discharges can be misleading, regardless of the source-modeling technique. In the case of primary generalized epilepsies, the MEG record typically shows a normal background

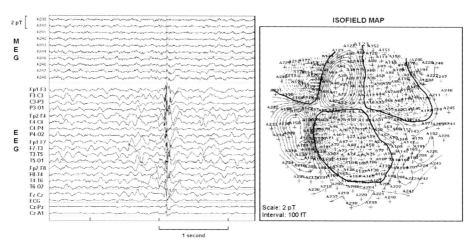

Fig. 14.4. Polyspike discharges preceding a generalized discharge. Following the leading spike over the left frontotemporal regions (F7-T3), a generalized discharge produced multiple dipolar maps (more evident over the left hemisphere) suggesting fast generalization. Filters: low frequency = 3 Hz; high frequency = 70 Hz. Amplitudes: MEG = 2 pT/cm; EEG = 50 μV/cm.

and generalized regular or irregular spike-and-wave and polyspike wave activity (Fig. 14.4). Isofield contour maps can indicate a focal onset preceding the generalized discharges, in agreement with the mild focal slowing and fragmented spikes with unilateral predominance. These findings can erroneously lead one to consider epilepsy as being focal when it is, indeed, generalized. Whether findings should be interpreted as a representation of the patterns of cortical spreading rather than of focal onset, though, remains controversial.

In secondary generalized epilepsies, diffuse slowing of the background activity associated with atypical generalized spike-wave complexes usually below 2.5 Hz occurs. Recordings typically show continuous high-amplitude generalized irregular discharges intermixed with multifocal spikes and sharp waves and the appearance of a chaotic background that, in some cases, can be interrupted by intermittent generalized attenuation.

The process of spike analysis and modeling, including the study of associated spatiotemporal maps, is time consuming and requires systematic training. After band-pass filtering (1 to 70 Hz is adequate) the MEG signals, one analyzes the interictal epileptiform discharges of MEG in three steps.

The first step entails selection of the epileptiform events. During this initial step, visual inspection of the simultaneous EEG recording is crucial for the classification of waveforms labeled as "epileptiform," since these events are yet to be defined based only on MEG features.

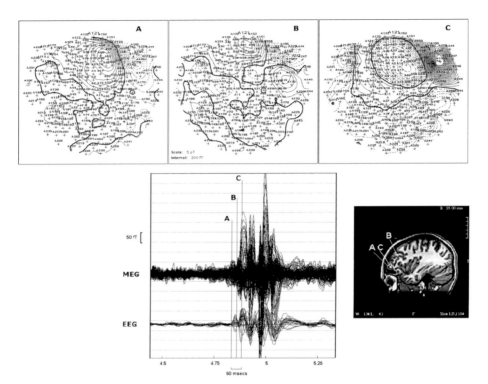

Fig. 14.5. Spatiotemporal analysis of interictal spike-and-waves. Top: isofield maps showing the pattern of onset: (A) rising period and (B) propagation in (C) a spike-and-wave discharge. Bottom: Note how the MEG deflections precede the EEG onset (8 to 10 ms). Filters: low frequency = 3 Hz; high frequency = 70 Hz. Amplitudes: MEG = 1 pT/cm; EEG = 50 μV/cm.

In the second step, after the time windows corresponding to each – or a highly representative sample – of the recorded epileptiform events have been identified, the spatiotemporal profile of the discharges is studied by looking at the isofield contour maps associated with the rising period of the wave or spike, the peak, and the pattern of propagation. These three stages of the discharge profile (see Fig. 14.5) may show different topographies and/or orientations in the contour maps that suggest the presence of a different source configuration for each of them. This step of the analysis is crucial for a detailed characterization of the irritative zone; one cannot substitute this step with an analysis of discharges only at the peak, where conditions of signal to noise are typically the best.

The third and final step requires modeling the intracranial sources that account for the recorded patterns and coregistration of the sources onto a structural image, typically an MRI. Features associated with the spatial distribution of the magnetic fields can modulate decisions regarding the algorithm with the most adequate fit, although consensus is that the ECD model can provide an accurate localization of interictal discharges in the majority of cases. Other decisions taken at this point can affect the validity of the solutions, i.e., characterization of background noise, selection of channel groups and local spheres for specific discharges. Once the resulting dipole sources are coregistered onto the patient's MRI (see Section I for a review of the process), characteristics like dipole orientation can provide significant insight into the actual structures responsible for the recorded epileptic discharges.

Ebersole [7, 8, 9] was the first to note that dipole orientation provided an essential clue for distinguishing foci in different temporal lobe regions. For instance, posterior temporal interictal spike dipoles with a vertical orientation correlate with sources in the lateral temporal cortex, while anterior temporal dipoles with a vertical orientation correlate with inferior and basal temporal cortex sources, and anterior temporal dipoles that are horizontal correlate with sources originating from the tip of the temporal lobe.

Ictal discharges

In most cases, MEG studies of patients with epilepsy are conducted on an outpatient basis, with patients maintained on their therapeutic level of antiepileptic medication. Therefore, ictal events are rare during MEG recordings, and movement artifacts often obscure the crucial brain activity. Consequently, ictal MEG is rarely documented in the literature. More often, 3 Hz spike-and-wave discharges can be documented in the absence of seizures, but the contribution of MEG can be controversial and limited in the characterization of epileptiform patterns preceding – or leading to – generalized discharges (see Fig. 14.6).

Most scalp EEG spikes are easily recognizable in simultaneous MEG recordings. Nonetheless, mismatching has frequently been reported for spikes in simultaneous scalp EEG and MEG evaluations, i.e., spikes found in MEG can be absent in scalp EEG and vice versa [5, 10–13]. In analyzing simultaneous scalp EEG and MEG, investigators commonly find morphological differences between coincident epileptiform events, such as in duration, sharpness, and shape, and attribute these differences to the physical conduction properties of electrical currents and to the orientation of the neuronal generation sites [4, 14–15].

A relevant study was conducted by Santiuste and colleagues to assess the sensitivity of whole-head MEG versus simultaneous depth-electrode EEG in the detection and localization of epileptic spikes [16]. An average of 100 spikes were found and analyzed for each of the 4 patients included in the study. Interictal MEG could correctly detect epileptiform events simultaneously recorded by depth electrodes, which had been implanted targeting ictal zones as determined

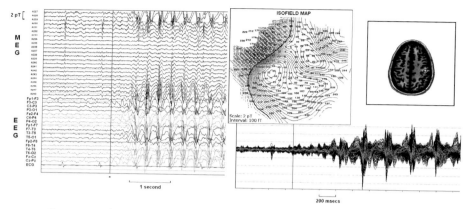

Fig. 14.6. Ictal MEG/EEG recordings in an adult (34 years old). Analysis of epileptiform events preceding generalized discharges suggests a contribution by the left perirolandic region to the irritative zone. The electrographic seizure was not accompanied by any symptoms. Left: simultaneous-tracing EEG/MEG showing the onset of the electrographic seizure. Center: isofield maps corresponding to the peak of one of the theta waves preceding the generalized discharges. Bottom right: MEG (black) and EEG (lighter lines) are collapsed showing the co-occurrence of the epileptiform patterns. Top right: source localization (left perirolandic) for the intracranial generator of the leading theta wave. Filters: low frequency = 3 Hz; high frequency = 70 Hz. Amplitudes: MEG = 1 pT/cm; EEG = 50 μV/cm.

by video-iEEG (intracranial EEG) monitoring (occipital lobe, amygdala, and hippocampus), in all 4 patients registered. Although not all iEEG spikes were detected by MEG, the ECD model of detected spikes accurately localized both to neocortical and deep ictal sources. Successful surgical resection of these areas further confirmed the MEG diagnoses, as all 4 patients remained seizure free (elapsed follow-up time was between 10 and 15 months). Based on these findings, the investigators concluded that interictal MEG's capacity to detect and localize the epileptogenic zone is comparable to that of depth electrodes when targeted to the convexity. When the epileptogenic zone is pinpointed to mesial structures of the brain, MEG spike localization and detection required epileptiform discharges with a higher amplitude and a wider distribution of the generators than was needed for discharges at the convexity. However, MEG still yields acceptable detectability and localization accuracy for clinical purposes.

15

Contributions of MEG to the surgical management of epilepsy – general considerations

Definitions

From a prospective study in newly diagnosed epilepsy cases, we find that 60% of patients become seizure-free on their first (47%) or second (13%) antiepileptic drug (AED) [17]. However, even when pharmacological treatment is effective, side effects and complications can severely limit success and general viability of the drug schedule. The 30% to 40% of patients who either do not respond to AED or suffer from side effects have only a small chance for subsequent remission with a second or third type of drug therapy [18]. For many of these patients, epilepsy surgery is a viable therapy option [19–22]. Optimal planning for such surgical procedures requires exact and reliable localization of the epileptogenic zone and determination of its spatial relationship to eloquent cortex. This zone is part of a broader network of abnormal activity. Within this network, different zones that have different functional significance for interictal and ictal epileptic activity can be distinguished.

A basic description of the epileptogenic zone was formulated by Penfield and Jasper in 1954 [23]. They defined the epileptogenic zone as the zone of actual seizure onset that had to be removed to achieve seizure freedom. The concept of Talairach and Bancaud extended this definition to include the early seizure-spread zone also [24]. A third view stated the large network hypothesis where all parts of the neuronal network are equally important and seizure freedom can be achieved by interruption of the network at any level [25–27]. Chauvel and coworkers [25] integrated the irritative and epileptogenic zone in a model focusing on the dynamic features of interictal activity and the identification of pacemakers. They reasoned that spatiotemporal analysis of hyperexcitability dynamics in the epileptic network also had to consider interictal propagation phenomena in the irritative network. According to Chauvel, primary and secondary irritative networks can be distinguished.

The concept of an epileptic focus as a network that is distributed and fuzzy in nature is more and more accepted. In many cases this network is concentrated in a small volume but can, in principle, be extended over larger areas without specific borders on a microscopic or even histological level. Diagnostic complexity increases with multiple foci, i.e., multiple subnetworks interconnected and distributed in the same or different lobes. Whereas small and condensed foci appear clinically as circumscribed lesions, larger networks cause diagnostic problems. Correct and accurate focus localization then may be difficult and might even cause misinterpretations.

Ictal MEG investigations

The recording time of MEG is limited to approximately 2 to 3 hours on average. Chances to record a seizure from a patient with rare or even moderately frequent seizures are therefore rather low, depending on patient selection. Even when an ictal event occurs, a number of technical problems limiting the diagnostic value of the recording exist. The main problems are poor signal quality, caused by muscle and movement artifacts, and movement of the head, resulting in subsequent invalidity of the coordinate system registered to the patient's head. The latter is likely to decrease in severity with recent developments that enable the detection – and even correction – of head movement by continually registering the head position. The resulting spatial information can then be used to correct mislocalization by taking the head position of the respective time interval into account or even correcting data by virtual projection to the sensor. Muscle artifacts, in turn, can be reduced by appropriate correction algorithms, however signal quality will remain limited. Therefore, analysis of clean data epochs early in the seizure, which are also more likely to reveal areas close to the seizure onset zone, is advisable. Regarding actual clinical value, several studies have shown good concordance between interictal and ictal MEG localizations [22, 28, 29]. However, findings of Eliashiv and colleagues [30] suggest that ictal MEG might be superior to interictal MEG, supporting opinions known from EEG analysis.

Comparison of interictal MEG with interictal and ictal EEG

Comparing localizations of interictal MEG and interictal EEG in patients with seizure-free surgical outcome, MEG and video-EEG localizations were similar in 32% and additional information could be obtained by MEG in 49% [31]. MEG hit the irritative zone more frequently than EEG [31, 32]. Oishi and coworkers [33] showed that single interictal clusters of localizations of interictal epileptic MEG activity correlated with invasively recorded seizure onset in 70%. Of 131 patients treated by epilepsy surgery, the correct lobe was localized in 89% [34].

Regarding spike yield, MEG and EEG are complementary. Knake and coworkers compared MEG and scalp EEG in a total of 70 patients and found spikes in MEG only in 12.9%, in EEG only in 2.9%, and in both MEG and EEG in 55.7% [35]. Another study by Scheler and associates compared MEG and EEG in 100 patients and found spikes in MEG only in 22%, spikes in EEG only in 7%, but 71% had spikes in both MEG and EEG [36].

When Papanicolaou and colleagues compared MEG findings with those from invasive EEG for 41 patients, they found correct MEG localizations in 56% and concordance with invasive EEG in 54% [37]. A study by Knowlton and coworkers of 49 patients revealed correct MEG localizations in 65% and invasive EEG localizations in 69.3% [38]. Otsubo and associates compared MEG spike localizations with electrocorticography (ECoG) and showed that localizations agreed in 12 of 12 patients [39]. Densely clustered interictal spike localizations correlated with the ability to localize seizure foci with ECoG in 11 of 16 patients, as reported by Mamelak and coworkers [40].

Surgical outcome

In patients with anterior temporal MEG spike localizations, surgical outcome was favorable after amygdala hippocampectomy [41]. Assaf and associates reported that patients with anterior vertical and anterior temporal horizontal dipoles became seizure free after undergoing an anterior mesial temporal resection or selective amygdala hippocampectomy [42]. Those with lateral vertical dipole orientations achieved seizure freedom after neocortical temporal surgery. When MEG localizations were represented as an ellipsoid volume and correlated with surgical outcome, the result was that the more an MEG-result ellipsoid covered a resection volume, the more seizure control was seen [43, 44].

Provocation methods

Methods used to increase the probability of spike recording – or recording of epileptiform activity – in clinical MEG are spike-inducing drugs, sleep deprivation, hyperventilation, photo/pattern stimulation, reduction of antiepileptic medication, or combinations of these.

Pharmacological spike activation has been studied for clonidine and methohexital [45]. Intravenously applied methohexital increased the frequency of focal epileptiform discharges in 8 of 13 patients; orally administered clonidine, in 9 of 14. Spike induction by methohexital has the advantage of shortening the recording time as compared to unprovoked recordings of interictal epileptiform discharges [46].

Spike activation by clonidine was compared to sleep deprivation in a study by Kettenman and coworkers investigating 22 patients [47]. About 67% of the patients showed increased spike activity after medication with clonidine, whereas sleep deprivation increased the number of spikes in 33%, and 29% of the patients showed no activation at all.

Sleep deprivation has been known for years to increase epileptic activity. Degen investigated the effect systematically from 127 EEGs taken while 102 epilepsy patients on anticonvulsant therapy were awake and asleep [48]. Epileptic activity increased from the 19% that was recorded on these patients' previous EEGs to 63% after sleep deprivation. Although the study was carried out using EEG, the results are probably also valid for MEG.

Some reports in the literature address anesthesia. Szmuk and colleagues found that MEG recorded while patients were under propofol anesthesia showed the least failure rate of interictal activity compared to MEG recorded from patients under anesthesia with other medication (e.g., midazolam) [49]. The study investigated only children; however, one can safely assume that the results are also true for adult epilepsy patients.

Inoue and colleagues studied changes in spike frequency when patients with photosensitivity and pattern sensitivity played electronic screen games during MEG recordings [50]. They found that spike frequency was induced in specific brain areas.

In some centers, application of chlorprothixene and doxylamine succinate before MEG measurement seems to provoke spikes by inducing drowsiness. Chlorprothixene has an additional epileptic activity-inducing effect. Systematic studies have not yet been performed however.

Source localization techniques in adult epilepsy

Common clinical practice for source localization of epileptic activity is single dipole analysis, which describes activity in terms of position, orientation, and amplitude of a single dipolar source. While rather simple compared to other available methods, dipole localization is effective as demonstrated by clinical studies [34, 40, 43, 44, 51–53]; results suggest that focal epileptic networks are mostly localized in a confined volume and can be adequately described by a single center of gravity.

More complex methods try to account for multiple or distributed sources and seem to be appropriate for describing extended and dynamic networks. While these methods are frequently used in cognitive research, their efficacy and validity in a clinical context has yet to be evaluated. In patients with extended epileptogenic networks and complex activity patterns, the use of such methods might prove beneficial [33, 54].

Alternative localization methods

In a study with 455 patients, no spike activity was detected during MEG investigations in approximately 30% [34]. In these patients, no diagnostic information could be obtained using standard MEG procedures. This percentage can be reduced – but not eliminated – by the application of provocation methods.

Current research is investigating alternatives to spike patterns that appear to be associated with the epileptic network. A promising alternative for focus localization seems to be slow-wave activity. Regarding lateralization, no disagreement has been shown between localization of trains of rhythmic slow waves and interictal spike activity in patients with mesial temporal lobe epilepsy (TLE) [55]. Slow-wave activity in patients with tumor-associated epilepsy occurs around the tumor [56]. The usefulness of low-frequency dipole density, together with localization of spike activity in patients with TLE, has been discussed by Fernandez and colleagues [57], who conclude that both slow-wave and spike analysis are valuable for presurgical epilepsy diagnostics in TLE patients. In a 2007 study [58], principal component analysis is used in an automated algorithm to localize slow-wave activity in epilepsy patients with focal epilepsies. Comparing clusters of spike and slow-wave dipole density localizations, the authors report a partial overlap of both. Maxima of slow-wave dipole density occur in the vicinity of the spike center of gravity, at distances ranging from 1 to 3 cm. Note that the automated algorithm used does not require any visual detection of slow-wave activity and is independent of spikes. Slow-wave localization results are obtained in both cryptogenic and symptomatic epilepsies, in TLE, and extratemporal lobe epilepsies (ETLE).

Another alternative to spike analysis is localization of general increases of spectral power, a technique that promises to yield information even in cases when dipole analysis fails [59]. Finally, investigation of high-frequency components as hypothetical surrogate markers of epilepsy might enable insights into basic mechanisms [60, 61].

16

MEG investigations in lesional epilepsies

A major domain of presurgical evaluation is the detection of lesions. About 80% of all surgical epilepsy patients present with a structural lesion on MRI; however, not all of these lesions are causally correlated with epilepsy. Determination of epileptogenicity is, therefore, essential. Functional modalities such as EEG and MEG play a crucial role. Iwasaki and colleagues found that if MEG localizations were congruent with a neocortical temporal lesion then lesionectomy was successful in controlling seizures [41].

In the case of multiple lesions, one has to decide which subset is relevant for seizure generation and which should consequently be subjected to surgical treatment. Pathologies commonly associated with ictal-onset regions are oligo-dendro glioma, ganglioglioma, focal cortical malformations, cavernoma with bleeding, or unilateral Ammon's horn sclerosis. More variable associations exist in the case of polymicrogyria, hemimegalencephaly, tuberous sclerosis, Sturge–Weber syndrome, and arachnoidal cysts.

Brain tumors

A considerable number of glioma patients show epileptic activity in the vicinity of tumor boundaries [62]. A close correlation between astrocytoma, gangli-oglioma, and leading spike activity within one centimeter of the tumor border was found in temporal lobe epilepsies by Stefan and colleagues [63]. Morioka and his associates showed that the localization of spike dipoles in patients with neurocytoma occurred around the tumor [64]. However, localizations of the hyperexcitable network were not always found in the whole circumference but can show predominant centers of gravity.

Vascular malformations

MEG spike localizations were congruent with spike localizations in intraoperative ECoG in patients with arteriovenous malformations [64]. In patients with single or multiple cavernomas, Stefan and colleagues demonstrated a correlation of lesion proximity to the irritative epileptic network and seizure outcome [65]. In addition to the hemosiderin fringe, neuronal cell loss and gliosis in the surrounding tissue of cavernomas may be responsible for the epileptogenesis in these symptomatic epilepsies. The resection of the cavernoma and hemosiderin fringe was shown to be a prognostic factor for seizure control [66].

Cortical malformations

Detection of cortical malformations can be challenging, as their extents can be barely recognizable by means of MRI. MEG-guided review of MRI images previously considered normal could detect subtle abnormalities with histopathological findings after successful epileptic surgery [67]. After MEG spike localization pointed to a distant region, reevaluation permitted detection of epileptogenic neocortical lesions on MRI that had been previously unidentified in 17.5% of the cases examined [68]. The location and extent of focal cortical dysplasia was predicted better by MEG than by extraoperative ECoG [55]. Several observations showed that the MEG-defined irritative network had to be removed to obtain seizure control in such cases, even if the irritative network extended beyond the borders of visible lesions in MRI [39, 69, 70]. In patients with bilateral EEG changes, MEG dipole clusters were confined to one hemisphere in the case of bilateral perisylvian syndromes [71]. Toulouse and colleagues used MEG to demonstrate involvement of both cortices in double cortex cases [72]. They showed that spikes initially involved the normal cortex and later the heterotopic cortex. In patients with tuberous sclerosis, MEG contributed to the recognition of the leading epileptogenic focus [73].

17

MEG investigations in nonlesional epilepsies

Nonlesional temporal lobe epilepsies (TLEs)

MEG is used to noninvasively differentiate between mesial and lateral neocortical epileptic regions in cases with nonlesional TLEs. In addition to dipole localizations, dipole orientations are being studied for diagnostic information. Anterior temporal vertical dipoles, according to Pataraia and coworkers [74], consistently localized to the mesial basal temporal compartments in the ipsilateral temporal lobe, whereas anterior horizontal dipoles localized more to the temporal pole and adjacent part of the lateral temporal lobe compartments and, in 50%, showed bitemporal spikes or seizure onsets. Surgical outcome after selective amygdala hippocampectomy was slightly better in patients with anterior temporal vertical dipoles. In other findings, anterior medial vertical dipoles were associated with mesial seizure onsets, while posterior lateral vertical dipoles occurred in patients with lateral or diffused seizure onsets [75, 76]. Comparisons of dipole orientations from data of different recordings will strongly depend on the choice of dipole source and volume conductor model. Simulations comparing different volume conductor models (spherical, 1- and 3-shell realistic BEM) demonstrated that differences of up to 90 degrees for the same spike patterns and analysis interval can occur, depending on tangentiality of the simulated source. Only the 3-shell realistic BEM was found to generate errors of less than 20 degrees with respect to the predefined simulated dipole orientation [77]. Results that differ from other findings might, therefore, be caused by differences in the analysis procedure rather than by actual (patho)physiology.

Extratemporal lobe epilepsies (ETLEs)

The frontal lobes account for 40% of the total cortex. For presurgical evaluation, these pose the problem of so-called "silent" areas producing no detectable ictal clinical signs during seizure onset. In addition, rapid spread through extensive connections adds to the diagnostic challenge, especially when structural imaging does not show any correlate. The time resolution of MEG allows us to localize and track onset and propagation of epileptic activity and investigate the spatial relationship to functional cortex, such as speech, motor, or somatosensory areas. Validity of the method has been demonstrated by various authors (e.g., by comparing MEG spike localizations with the results of invasive recordings) [32, 34, 39, 51, 78–85]. In cases with normal MRI findings, irritative networks could be identified by means of MEG [84] and can lead to the subsequent identification of subtle lesions, such as cortical malformations [86]. Source-localization results in nonlesional cases can thus provide additional information for reevaluation of previous MRIs or allow for focused imaging (e.g., using surface coils). Invasive recordings also benefit significantly from optimized placement of electrodes based on MEG findings and are more likely to identify seizure onset and irritative zones [84]. Removal of these zones frequently results in postoperative seizure control [39, 43, 44].

18

Pediatric nonlesional epilepsy surgery

Overview

Pediatric epilepsy surgery – and the candidates referred for evaluation of pediatric epilepsy – are distinctly different from adult epilepsy surgery and adult referral candidates [87, 88]. Additionally, the goals of epilepsy surgery in children may include objectives other than seizure freedom (e.g., developmental progression). A recent survey conducted by the Pediatric Epilepsy Surgery Subcommission of the International League Against Epilepsy (ILAE) revealed that the most common final operation was lobar and focal resection of the frontal and temporal lobes and that the majority of all children operated on had an apparent lesion on MRI [87]. Identification of a focal lesion on MRI increases the chance of delineating a focal resectable epileptic network. Postsurgical seizure freedom is related to the resection of the correct epileptic zone. Studies in adults have found better postsurgical outcome for MRI-positive patients as opposed to MRI-negative patients [89]. Though the currently available MRI may not identify a focal brain lesion, histopathological examination of the resected tissue often demonstrates the specific pathology [90, 91]. Hence the term "nonlesional" may be a misnomer.

However, in the ILAE survey a small group of children with no or subtle MRI findings (nonlesional MRI) did undergo epilepsy surgery [87]. Few studies were available in the literature that evaluated postsurgical seizure freedom in children with intractable localization-related epilepsy and normal or nonspecific MRI findings [90–92]. Case selection criteria and expertise of the epilepsy center determined the postsurgical outcome in such children.

No accurate estimate of the prevalence of normal MRI findings in children with intractable epilepsy who are potential surgical candidates is available. The majority of children with normal MRIs would seem not to be surgical candidates during presurgical evaluation. However, the weight given to a normal or nonspecific MRI depends on the case selection criteria adopted by the epilepsy center, since each center decides surgical candidacy in patients with normal MRI findings based on their own presurgical evaluation modalities [91]. Lee and colleagues reported good postsurgical seizure outcome in 80% of 89 patients (adult and pediatric) with cryptogenic neocortical epilepsy [93]. In a group of 24 adult and pediatric patients, Chapman and coworkers reported 37% seizure freedom and more than 90% seizure reduction in 75% of patients [90]. Only two series are exclusively pediatric. Paolicchi and colleagues reported a higher overall percentage of postsurgical seizure freedom (51%) in 35 children with nonlesional epilepsy [92], whereas RamachandranNair and coworkers reported good outcome in 77% (seizure free: 36%) in 22 children [91]. Nine of 11 children – only one patient had a focal MRI lesion – in the series studied by Minassian and associates became either seizure free or had a greater than 90% reduction in seizures after surgery, with a mean follow-up of 24 months [82].

Children with a nonlesional MRI – defined here as no apparent lesion or only a subtle lesion on a good quality 1.5 tesla (T) or 3T MRI with specific epilepsy sequences – are the subject of this chapter. The chapter will focus on four situations where MEG testing for epilepsy dipoles is helpful in the evaluation of pediatric patients for epilepsy surgery.

Lobectomy or topectomy candidates

Early prospective, comparative studies demonstrated the utility of MEG in patients – children and adults – evaluated for epilepsy surgery [32]. Subsequent comparative studies from the same center evaluated children and adults with lesional or nonlesional refractory partial epilepsy and sought to determine which patient subgroup might benefit the most from undergoing preoperative MEG testing [31, 37]. Historically, the presence of a lesion on an MRI has been one of the most important factors in determining the outcome of the epilepsy surgery evaluation (see Fig. 18.1) [87]. In a series of 82 consecutive patients, the contribution of MEG was greatest in patients with inconsistently localizing scalp video-EEG results [31]. While this study included children, the data were not further analyzed based on the influence of an MRI lesion [31, 37]. However, the study suggested that MEG may be an important diagnostic tool in children who have nonlocalizing EEGs – typically, nonlesional MRIs – and refractory partial epilepsy.

Whole-head MEG testing is used in the evaluation of children with nonlesional refractory epilepsy. The method that follows is an example of procedures currently in use at one center (the Hospital for Sick Children in Toronto, Canada) to map the irritative zone.

MEG and EEG are recorded simultaneously with a band-pass filter of 3 to 70 Hz and notch filter of 60 Hz. MEG epileptic discharges – spikes and sharp waves (referred to as spikes) – are visually identified on the MEG recordings and

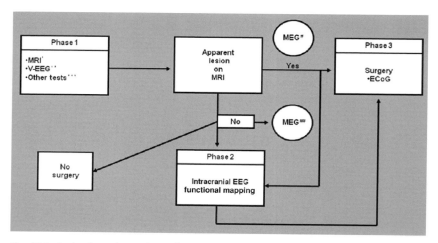

Fig. 18.1. Evaluation schema for pediatric epilepsy surgery.

cross-referenced with the EEG recording. A single moving dipole analysis with a single-shell, whole-head spherical model is applied to the MEG data. MEG spike dipoles are defined for each spike using a single dipole fit starting from the earliest phase of each spike with the criteria of a residual error of less than 30%. The MEG spike dipole sources are mapped onto the MRI (T1-WI; 2 mm thickness, no skip) pixels with a software program (MARK VOXEL). The MEG spike dipole source distributions are then classified into four groups by number and density: Class I (clusters), consisting of 20 or more spike sources with 1 cm or less between adjacent sources; Class II (small clusters), consisting of 6 to 19 spike sources with 1 cm or less between adjacent sources; Class III (scatters), consisting of less than 6 spike sources regardless of the distance between sources, or spike sources with greater than 1 cm between sources regardless of the number of sources in a group; and Class IV (no MEG spike dipole source) [94]. The MRI data coregistered with pixels of dipoles are transferred (via DICOM 3.0) to a workstation (General Electric Advantage Windows 3.1) and from there transferred to a picture-archiving and communications system. A seeded-threshold method is used on specialized software (ISG Allegro 3-D software) to create a 3-D shaded-surface display of the skin surface, the brain surface, the lesion, if any, and the dipoles of the epileptic discharges and SEFs. The 2-D and 3-D data sets are loaded onto a neurosurgical neuronavigation system (Zeiss/SNN Neurosurgical Navigational System). This frameless stereotaxy system is used in the operating-room setting to localize the MEG data directly onto the patient's brain. Surface registration correlates the images with the surgical system (see Fig. 18.2) [95]. Extraoperative intracranial video-EEG monitoring from sub-dural grid electrodes is performed before epilepsy surgery. The subdural grid is

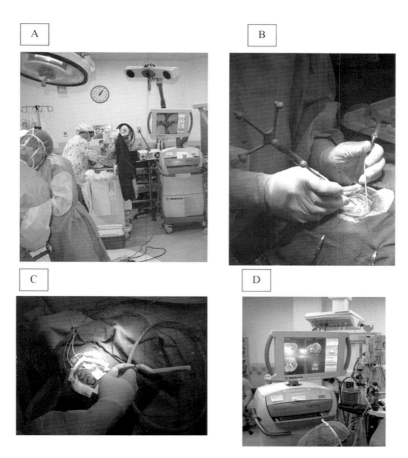

Fig. 18.2. Neuronavigational system (Medtronic Stealth System TREON plus) with MRI and MEG data loaded and being used (A) in the operating room; (B) to coregister brain surface with MRI and MEG images (standard system with head in frame below the drapes); (C) to coregister brain surface and subdural strip electrodes, using infrared, frameless system (no head frame, which allows use in young children whose skull cannot support the frame system, as seen in images A and B); (D) to coregister brain surface with MRI and MEG image (infrared system with no frame for head).

constructed based on the 3-D MRIs, interictal and ictal scalp EEG results, MEG spike dipole sources, MEG-somatosensory evoked-response source locations, and clinical symptoms [94].

Two studies have helped to define the role of MEG in nonlesional, partial-onset, refractory pediatric epilepsy [82, 91]. As a result, MEG has been added to the evaluation protocol for these patients in some institutions and has altered the

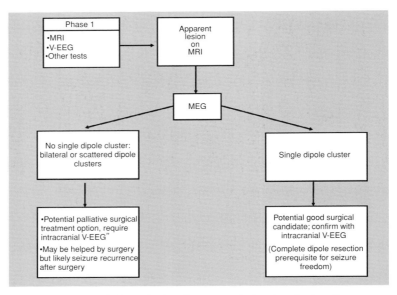

Fig. 18.3. Magnetoencephalography (MEG) use in nonlesional pediatric epilepsy.

hospitals' diagnostic paradigm (see 18.1, expanded in Fig. 18.3, at The Hospital for Sick Children). In the first study, MEG was performed in 11 children with intractable, nonlesional, extratemporal, localization-related epilepsy [82]. They studied the concordance of the anatomical location of interictal MEG spike foci with the location of ictal-onset zones identified by invasive ictal intracranial EEG recordings in children undergoing evaluation for epilepsy surgery. Based on the invasive monitoring data, all children had excision of – or multiple subpial transactions through – ictal-onset cortex and surrounding irritative zones. In all children, the anatomical location of the somatosensory hand area, determined by functional mapping through the subdural grid, was the same as that delineated by MEG.

In 10 of the patients, the anatomical location of the epileptiform discharges, as determined by MEG, corresponded to the ictal-onset zone established by ictal intracranial recordings [82]. Additionally, 9 of the 11 patients had a greater than 90% seizure reduction or complete seizure freedom after surgery. This preliminary study revealed MEG to be an accurate and powerful tool in the presurgical evaluation of children with refractory, nonlesional, extratemporal epilepsy and suggested three important findings related to the dipole clusters obtained by MEG: (1) a single discrete cluster predicted the best surgical outcome (seizure freedom); (2) the number and extent of dipole clusters has important prognostic implications; (3) complete resection of the dipole cluster

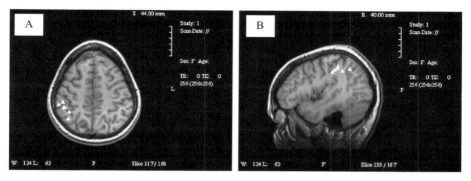

Fig. 18.4. (a) Single dipole cluster, small area; (b) Single dipole cluster (same patient as in (a)).

is usually necessary to achieve seizure freedom. (A complete resection could be limited by the presence of eloquent cortex.)

In the second study, RamachandranNair and colleagues investigated the predictors of postsurgical seizure freedom in 22 children with refractory epilepsy and normal or nonfocal MRI findings. MEG dipole clusters were located in a single hemisphere in 18 children [91]. Three children had bilateral MEG dipole clusters and 1 child had only scattered dipoles. Seventeen children (77%) had good postsurgical outcomes (defined as Engel class IIIA or better), and 8 of the 17 (36%) were seizure free. MEG dipole clusters were present in the region of final resection in 18 children. Thirteen of these children (72.2%) had good postsurgical seizure outcomes; including 8 who were seizure free. All the children with postsurgical seizure freedom had the MEG dipole cluster in the final resection area (see Fig. 18.4). In 17 cases with good postsurgical outcome, the MEG dipole cluster correctly localized the resection area in 13, interictal EEG in 7, and ictal scalp video-EEG in 6. The absence of an MEG dipole cluster located exclusively within the region of final resection had 100% negative predictive value with respect to postsurgical seizure freedom since postsurgical seizure freedom was obtained in none of the 4 children who had bilateral MEG dipole clusters or only scattered dipoles (see Fig. 18.5). Conversely, all children who had postsurgical seizure freedom also had an MEG dipole cluster confined to the resection area. The ictal-onset zone was localized in the 3 children who had bilateral MEG dipole clusters after two-stage intracranial extraoperative monitoring (2 children) or simultaneous bilateral recording (1 child). However, surgery failed in all 4 of these children. These findings led to two interesting conclusions: the presence of an MEG dipole cluster confined to the resection area is a prerequisite for postsurgical seizure freedom [87], and the absence of an MEG dipole cluster or the presence of bilateral MEG dipole clusters or scatters may predict seizure recurrence following epilepsy surgery [88, 91].

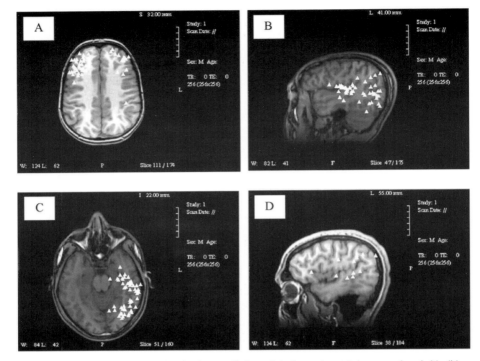

Fig. 18.5. (a) Bilateral dipole clusters (bifrontal, independent, right more than left); (b) Scattered, unilateral dipoles (left hemisphere: temporal, parietal); (c) Scattered, unilateral dipoles (axial view, same patient as in b); (d) Scattered, unilateral dipoles (left hemisphere has paucity of clustered and scattered dipoles).

As a result of the larger RamachandranNair study, the role of the MEG dipole cluster has been included in the patient evaluation and preoperative prognostic discussions with families at some hospitals (see Fig. 18.3) [53, 91]. Additional MEG diagnostic studies (see Fig. 18.6) can be performed based on the suspected epileptogenic zone and location of MEG clusters. This information adds to the risk–benefit discussion with families and assists in surgical planning.

Corpus callosotomy

Corpus callosotomy is a useful surgical procedure for intractable seizures in children who are not candidates for focal resective surgery. This procedure is used primarily in children with nonlesional MRI who have frequent drop attacks (generalized atonic or tonic seizures) or generalized tonic–clonic seizures.

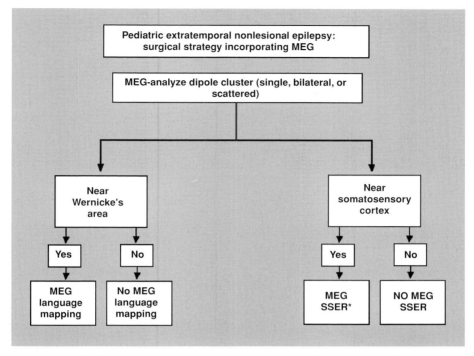

Fig. 18.6. Contribution of MEG to the presurgical evaluation of pediatric nonlesional epilepsy.

Typically, affected children have a high seizure burden with resultant multiple abrasions, tooth avulsions, fractures and lacerations due to falls. Historically, anterior two-thirds, two-stage procedures, and complete section of the corpus callosum have been performed, depending on the patient's level of cognitive function and dominant hand – and suspected dominant hemisphere for speech. Today, however, most recommend a complete or near-complete callosal section in patients with mental retardation – a common finding in the majority of candidates [96, 97].

MEG may assist in the evaluation of these children for callosotomy in the following ways: (1) in children who have mild cognitive impairment or normal cognitive function, MEG can confirm the colocalization of language function and dominant hand to the same hemisphere. Since complete callosotomy is contraindicated for patients with hand dominance in one hemisphere and language dominance in the other [98] and these patients may be at higher risk for cognitive and behavioral problems, the MEG information will help plan the staging of the procedure and potential rehabilitation; (2) preliminary data

suggest the interhemispheric time difference of bilateral synchronized discharges measured by MEG may have prognostic implications [99]. Those
discharges that demonstrate a rapid interhemispheric time difference (<20
ms) on MEG correlate with a more dramatic reduction in drop attacks. Longer
interhemispheric time differences (>80 ms) suggest polysynaptic nontranscal-
losal pathways and a poorer response to callosotomy; (3) MEG characterization of the interictal bisynchronous discharges, detected by scalp EEG, may
have prognostic implications. Children whose scalp EEG findings are bisynchronous, but whose MEG testing reveals left or independent right-leading
onset, with accompanying symptomatic generalized epilepsy, are not candidates for focal resection and often develop independent, hemispheric partial-
onset seizures after surgery. This information is helpful in counseling the family
preoperatively (i.e., unilateral, extratemporal onset with rapid secondary generalization that would suggest focal resection is not present), and postoperatively (i.e., to watch for independent left or right body seizures, and track each
type).

Nonlesional refractory status epilepticus

A single, preliminary report of five children with refractory status epilepticus addresses the role of MEG in localizing the epileptogenic zone for surgical treatment [100]. Two of the five children had normal MRIs at presentation and recordings of interictal MEG spike sources, and one child had ictal
MEG spike sources. Both underwent anterior temporal lobectomy, and while
not seizure free, experienced enough improvement to have their high-dose
suppressive therapy stopped and could be discharged on oral AEDs. These
results highlight another potential diagnostic role of MEG in this select patient
group.

Conclusion

MEG, using a whole-head system, is now a critical diagnostic tool in the evaluation of children with refractory nonlesional epilepsy who are being considered for epilepsy surgery. The utility of MEG in epilepsy surgery evaluation
is dependent on the child having epileptiform discharges (dipoles) during the
40- to 60-minute study. The location and extent of the dipoles provide crucial
information to surgical planning and provide important prognostic information. Additionally, intractable, nonlesional epilepsy in children typically has
an extratemporal origin, often requiring functional mapping with MEG at the
same time as the dipole study. The entire MEG study must be carefully planned
(e.g., language mapping may be performed first while the child is awake, then

epilepsy dipoles and somatosensory evoked responses could be obtained with the child asleep). Coregistration of all this data on the same magnetic source image is then performed. The data can then be retrieved in the operating room using a frameless, stereotaxic neuronavigational system to guide surgery, to perform intraoperative mapping (for confirmation of MEG findings), or to place electrodes.

References

1. Berger, H. Uber das Electrenkephalogramm des Menschen. *Arch Psychiatr Nervenkr* 1929; **87**: 527–570.
2. International Federation of Societies for Clinical Neurophysiology. A glossary of terms most commonly used by clinical electroencephalographers. *Electroencephalogr Clin Neurophysiol* 1974; **37**(5): 538–548.
3. Zijlmans M, Huiskamp GM, Leijten FSS, van der Meij WM, Wieneke G, van Huffelen AC. Modality-specific spike identification in simultaneous magnetoencephalography/electroencephalography. *J Clin Neurophysiol* 2002; **19**: 183–191.
4. Fernandes JM, Martins da Silva A, Huiskamp GM, *et al.* What does an epileptiform spike look like in MEG? Comparison between coincident EEG and MEG spikes. *J Clin Neurophysiol* 2005; **22**: 68–73.
5. Iwasaki M, Pestana E, Burgess RC, Luders HO, Shamoto H, Nakasato N. Detection of epileptiform activity by human interpreters: blinded comparison between EEG and MEG. *Epilepsia* 2005; **46**: 59–68.
6. Nowak R, Santiuste M, Russi A, *et al.* Toward a definition of MEG spike: parametric description of spikes recorded simultaneously by MEG and depth electrodes. *Biomag 2008. Biomagnetism: Transdisciplinary Research and Exploration; Proceedings of Sixteenth International Conference on Biomagnetism*; 2008 August 25–29; Sapporo, Japan. 2008.
7. Ebersole JS. Non-invasive localization of the epileptogenic focus by EEG dipole modeling. *Acta Neurol Scand Suppl* 1994; **152**: 20–28.
8. Ebersole JS. Clinical application of voltage topography and source localization in partial epilepsy. In: Angeleri F, Butler S, Giaquinto S, Majkowski J, eds. *Analysis of the Electrical Activity of the Brain.* Chichester, UK: John Wiley & Sons. 1997; 263–270.
9. Ebersole JS. EEG/MEG dipole modeling. In: Engel J, Pedley T, eds. *Comprehensive Epileptology.* Philadephia: Lippincott–Raven. 1997; 919–936.
10. Iwasaki M, Nakasato N, Shamoto H, Yoshimoto T. Focal magnetoencephalographic spikes in the superior temporal plane undetected by scalp EEG. *J Clin Neurosci* 2003; **10**: 236–238.
11. Lin YY, Shih YH, Hsieh JC, *et al.* Magnetoencephalographic yield of interictal spikes in temporal lobe epilepsy. Comparison with scalp EEG recordings. *NeuroImage* 2003; **19**: 1115–1126.
12. Park HM, Nakasato N, Iwasaki M, Shamoto H, Tominaga T, Yoshimoto T. Comparison of magnetoencephalographic spikes with and without concurrent

electroencephalographic spikes in extratemporal epilepsy. *Tohoku J Exp Med* 2004; **203**: 165–174.

13. Kirsch HE, Mantle M, Nagarajan SS. Concordance between routine interictal magnetoencephalography and simultaneous scalp electroencephalography in a sample of patients with epilepsy. *J Clin Neurophysiol* 2007; **24**: 215–231.

14. Merlet I, Paetau R, García-Larrea L, Uutela K, Granström ML, Mauguière F. Apparent asynchrony between interictal electric and magnetic spikes. *Neuroreport* 1997; **24**: 1071–1076.

15. Parra J, Kalitzin SN, da Silva FH. Magnetoencephalography: an investigational tool or a routine clinical technique? *Epilepsy Behav* 2004; **5**: 277–285.

16. Santiuste M, Nowak R, Russi A, *et al.* Simultaneous magnetoencephalography and intracranial EEG registration: technical and clinical aspects. *J Clin Neurophysiol* 2008 (in press).

17. Kwan P, Brodie MJ. Early identification of refractory epilepsy. *N Engl J Med* 2000; **342:** 314–319.

18. Brodie MJ, Kwan P. Staged approach to epilepsy management. *Neurology* 2002; **58**(8Suppl 5): S2–S8.

19. Clusmann H, Kral T, Schramm J. Present practice and perspective of evaluation and surgery for temporal lobe epilepsy. *Zentralbl Neurochir* 2006; **67**: 165–182.

20. Cohen-Gadol AA, Wilhelmi BG, Collignon F, *et al.* Long-term outcome of epilepsy surgery among 399 patients with nonlesional seizure foci including mesial temporal lobe sclerosis. *J Neurosurg* 2006; **104**: 513–524.

21. Stern JM. Overview of treatment guidelines for epilepsy. *Curr Treatm Options Neurol* 2006; **8**: 280–288.

22. Tang L, Mantle M, Ferrari P, *et al.* Consistency of interictal and ictal onset localization using magnetoencephalography in patients with partial epilepsy. *J Neurosurg* 2003; **98**: 837–845.

23. Penfield W, Jasper H. *Epilepsy and the Functional Anatomy of the Human Brain.* Boston: Little Brown, 1954.

24. Talairach J, Bancaud J. Lesion, "irritative" zone and epileptogenic focus. *Confin Neurol* 1966; **27**: 91–94.

25. Chauvel P, Buser P, Badier JM, Liegeois-Chauvel C, Marquis P, Bancaud J. The "epileptogenic zone" in humans: representation of intercritical events by spatio-temporal maps. *Rev Neurol* (Paris) 1987; **143**: 443–450.

26. Sutherling WW, Barth DS. Neocortical propagation in temporal lobe spike foci on magnetoencephalography and electroencephalography. *Ann Neurol* 1989; **25**: 373–381.

27. Stefan H, Schneider S, Abraham-Fuchs K, *et al.* The neocortico to mesio-basal limbic propagation of focal epileptic activity during the spike-wave complex. *Electroencephalogr Clin Neurophysiol* 1991; **79**: 1–10.

28. Assaf BA, Karkar KM, Laxer KD, *et al.* Ictal magnetoencephalography in temporal and extratemporal lobe epilepsy. *Epilepsia* 2003; **44**: 1320–1327.

29. Tilz C, Hummel C, Kettenmann B, Stefan H. Ictal onset localization of epileptic seizures by magnetoencephalography. *Acta Neurol Scand* 2002; **106**: 190–195.

30. Eliashiv DS, Elsas SM, Squires K, Fried I, Engel J, Jr. Ictal magnetic source imaging as a localizing tool in partial epilepsy. *Neurology* 2002; **59**: 1600–1610.

31. Pataraia E, Simos PG, Castillo EM, *et al.* Does magnetoencephalography add to scalp video-EEG as a diagnostic tool in epilepsy surgery? *Neurology* 2004; **62**: 943–948.

32. Wheless JW, Willmore LJ, Breier JI, *et al.* A comparison of magnetoencephalography, MRI, and V-EEG in patients evaluated for epilepsy surgery. *Epilepsia* 1999; **40**: 931–941.

33. Oishi M, Otsubo H, Iida K, *et al.* Preoperative simulation of intracerebral epileptiform discharges: synthetic aperture magnetometry virtual sensor analysis of interictal magnetoencephalography data. *J Neurosurg* 2006; **105**: 41–49.

34. Stefan H, Hummel C, Scheler G, *et al.* Magnetic brain source imaging of focal epileptic activity: a synopsis of 455 cases. *Brain* 2003; **126**: 2396–2405.

35. Knake S, Halgren E, Shiraishi H, *et al.* The value of multichannel MEG and EEG in the presurgical evaluation of 70 epilepsy patients. *Epilepsy Res* 2006; **69**: 80–86.

36. Scheler G, Fischer MJ, Genow A, *et al.* Spatial relationship of source localizations in patients with focal epilepsy: comparison of MEG and EEG with a three spherical shells and a boundary element volume conductor model. *Hum Brain Mapp* 2007; **28**: 315–322.

37. Papanicolaou AC, Pataraia E, Billingsley-Marshall R, *et al.* Toward the substitution of invasive electroencephalography in epilepsy surgery. *J Clin Neurophysiol* 2005; **22**: 231–237.

38. Knowlton RC, Elgavish R, Howell J, *et al.* Magnetic source imaging versus intracranial electroencephalogram in epilepsy surgery: a prospective study. *Ann Neurol* 2006; **59**: 835–842.

39. Otsubo H, Ochi A, Elliott I, *et al.* MEG predicts epileptic zone in lesional extrahippocampal epilepsy: 12 pediatric surgery cases. *Epilepsia* 2001; **42**: 1523–1530.

40. Mamelak AN, Lopez N, Akhtari M, Sutherling WW. Magnetoencephalography-directed surgery in patients with neocortical epilepsy. *J Neurosurg* 2002; **97**: 865–873.

41. Iwasaki M, Nakasato N, Shamoto H, *et al.* Surgical implications of neuromagnetic spike localization in temporal lobe epilepsy. *Epilepsia* 2002; **43**: 415–424.

42. Assaf BA, Karkar KM, Laxer KD, *et al.* Magnetoencephalography source localization and surgical outcome in temporal lobe epilepsy. *Clin Neurophysiol* 2004; **115**: 2066–2076.

43. Fischer MJ, Scheler G, Stefan H. Utilization of magnetoencephalography results to obtain favourable outcomes in epilepsy surgery. *Brain* 2005; **128**: 153–157.

44. Genow A, Hummel C, Scheler G, *et al.* Epilepsy surgery, resection volume and MSI localization in lesional frontal lobe epilepsy. *NeuroImage* 2004; **21**: 444–449.

45. Kirchberger K, Schmitt H, Hummel C, *et al.* Clonidine- and methohexital-induced epileptiform discharges detected by magnetoencephalography (MEG) in patients with localization-related epilepsies. *Epilepsia* 1998; **39**: 1104–1112.

46. Brockhaus A, Lehnertz K, Wienbruch C, *et al.* Possibilities and limitations of magnetic source imaging of methohexital-induced epileptiform patterns in temporal lobe epilepsy patients. *Electroencephalogr Clin Neurophysiol* 1997; **102**: 423–436.

47. Kettenmann B, Feichtinger M, Tilz C, Kaltenhauser M, Hummel C, Stefan H. Comparison of clonidine to sleep deprivation in the potential to induce spike or sharp-wave activity. *Clin Neurophysiol* 2005; **116**: 905–912.

48. Degen R. A study of the diagnostic value of waking and sleep EEGs after sleep deprivation in epileptic patients on anticonvulsive therapy. *Electroencephalogr Clin Neurophysiol* 1980; **49**: 577–584.

49. Szmuk P, Kee S, Pivalizza EG, Warters RD, Abramson DC, Ezri T. Anaesthesia for magnetoencephalography in children with intractable seizures. *Paediatr Anaesth* 2003; **13**: 811–817.

50. Inoue Y, Fukao K, Araki T, Yamamoto S, Kubota H, Watanabe Y. Photosensitive and nonphotosensitive electronic screen game-induced seizures. *Epilepsia* 1999; **40** (Suppl 4): 8–16.

51. Knowlton RC, Laxer KD, Aminoff MJ, Roberts TP, Wong ST, Rowley HA. Magnetoencephalography in partial epilepsy: clinical yield and localization accuracy. *Ann Neurol* 1997; **42**: 622–631.

52. Oishi M, Otsubo H, Kameyama S, *et al*. Epileptic spikes: magnetoencephalography versus simultaneous electrocorticography. *Epilepsia* 2002; **43**: 1390–1395.

53. Oishi M, Kameyama S, Masuda H, *et al*. Single and multiple clusters of magnetoencephalographic dipoles in neocortical epilepsy: significance in characterizing the epileptogenic zone. *Epilepsia* 2006; **47**: 355–364.

54. Xiao Z, Xiang J, Holowka S, *et al*. Volumetric localization of epileptic activities in tuberous sclerosis using synthetic aperture magnetometry. *Pediatr Radiol* 2006; **36**: 16–21.

55. Ishibashi H, Simos PG, Castillo EM, *et al*. Detection and significance of focal, interictal, slow-wave activity visualized by magnetoencephalography for localization of a primary epileptogenic region. *J Neurosurg* 2002; **96**: 724–730.

56. Baayen JC, de Jongh A, Stam CJ, *et al*. Localization of slow wave activity in patients with tumor-associated epilepsy. *Brain Topogr* 2003; **16**: 85–93.

57. Fernandez A, de Sola RG, Amo C, *et al*. Dipole density of low-frequency and spike magnetic activity: a reliable procedure in presurgical evaluation of temporal lobe epilepsy. *J Clin Neurophysiol* 2004; **21**: 254–266.

58. Kaltenhauser M, Scheler G, Rampp S, Paulini A, Stefan H. Spatial intralobar correlation of spike and slow wave activity localisations in focal epilepsies: a MEG analysis. *NeuroImage* 2007; **34**: 1466–1472.

59. Xiang J, Holowka S, Qiao H, *et al*. Automatic localization of epileptic zones using magnetoencephalography. *Neurol Clin Neurophysiol* 2004; **2004**: 98.

60. da Silva FH, Gomez JP, Velis DN, Kalitzin S. Phase clustering of high frequency EEG: MEG components. *Clin EEG Neurosci* 2005; **36**: 306–310.

61. Rampp S, Stefan H. Fast activity as a surrogate marker of epileptic network function? *Clin Neurophysiol* 2006; **117**: 2111–2117.

62. Patt S, Steenbeck J, Hochstetter A, *et al*. Source localization and possible causes of interictal epileptic activity in tumor-associated epilepsy. *Neurobiol Dis* 2000; **7**: 260–269.

63. Stefan H, Schuler P, Abraham-Fuchs K, *et al*. Magnetic source localization and morphological changes in temporal lobe epilepsy: comparison of MEG/EEG, ECoG and volumetric MRI in presurgical evaluation of operated patients. *Acta Neurol Scand Suppl* 1994; **152**: 83–88.

64. Morioka T, Nishio S, Shigeto H, *et al*. Surgical management of intractable epilepsy associated with cerebral neurocytoma. *Neurol Res* 2000; **22**: 449–456.

65. Stefan H, Scheler G, Hummel C, *et al.* Magnetoencephalography (MEG) predicts focal epileptogenicity in cavernomas. *J Neurol Neurosurg Psychiatry* 2004; **75**: 1309–1313.

66. Hammen T, Romstock J, Dorfler A, Kerling F, Buchfelder M, Stefan H. Prediction of postoperative outcome with special respect to removal of hemosiderin fringe: a study in patients with cavernous haemangiomas associated with symptomatic epilepsy. *Seizure* 2007; **16**: 248–253.

67. Zhang W, Simos PG, Ishibashi H, *et al.* Multimodality neuroimaging evaluation improves the detection of subtle cortical dysplasia in seizure patients. *Neurol Res* 2003; **25**: 53–57.

68. Moore KR, Funke ME, Constantino T, Katzman GL, Lewine JD. Magnetoencephalographically directed review of high-spatial-resolution surface-coil MR images improves lesion detection in patients with extratemporal epilepsy. *Radiology* 2002; **225**: 880–887.

69. Morioka T, Nishio S, Ishibashi H, *et al.* Intrinsic epileptogenicity of focal cortical dysplasia as revealed by magnetoencephalography and electrocorticography. *Epilepsy Res* 1999; **33**: 177–187.

70. Bast T, Oezkan O, Rona S, *et al.* EEG and MEG source analysis of single and averaged interictal spikes reveals intrinsic epileptogenicity in focal cortical dysplasia. *Epilepsia* 2004; **45**: 621–631.

71. Tanaka M, Yamada K, Watanabe Y, *et al.* Electroclinical and magnetoencephalographic analysis of epilepsy in patients with congenital bilateral perisylvian syndrome. *Epilepsia* 2000; **41**: 1584–1591.

72. Toulouse P, Agulhon C, Taussig D, *et al.* Magnetoencephalographic studies of two cases of diffuse subcortical laminar heterotopia or so-called double cortex. *NeuroImage* 2003; **19**: 1251–1259.

73. Peresson M, Lopez L, Narici L, Curatolo P. Magnetic source imaging and reactivity to rhythmical stimulation in tuberous sclerosis. *Brain Dev* 1998; **20**: 512–518.

74. Pataraia E, Lindinger G, Deecke L, Mayer D, Baumgartner C. Combined MEG/EEG analysis of the interictal spike complex in mesial temporal lobe epilepsy. *NeuroImage* 2005; **24**: 607–614.

75. Baumgartner C, Pataraia E, Lindinger G, Deecke L. Magnetoencephalography in focal epilepsy. *Epilepsia* 2000; **41**: 39–47.

76. Ebersole JS. Non-invasive pre-surgical evaluation with EEG/MEG source analysis. *Electroencephalogr Clin Neurophysiol Suppl* 1999; **50**: 167–174.

77. Crouzeix A, Yvert B, Bertrand O, Pernier J. An evaluation of dipole reconstruction accuracy with spherical and realistic head models in MEG. *Clin Neurophysiol* 1999; **110**: 2176–2188.

78. Paetau R, Kajola M, Karhu J, *et al.* Magnetoencephalographic localization of epileptic cortex–impact on surgical treatment. *Ann Neurol* 1992; **32**: 106–109.

79. Nakasato N, Levesque MF, Barth DS, Baumgartner C, Rogers, RL, Sutherling WW. Comparison of MEG, EEG, and ECoG source localization in neocortical partial epilepsy in humans. *Electroencephalogr Clin Neurophysiol* 1994; **91**: 171–178.

80. Smith JR, Gallen C, Orrison W, *et al.* Role of multichannel magnetoencephalography in the evaluation of ablative seizure surgery candidates. *Stereotact Funct Neurosurg* 1994; **62**: 238–244.

81. Mohamed IS, Otsubo H, Ochi A, *et al.* Utility of magnetoencephalography in the evaluation of recurrent seizures after epilepsy surgery. *Epilepsia* 2007; **48**: 2150–2159.

82. Minassian BA, Otsubo H, Weiss S, Elliott I, Rutka JT, Snead OC, III Magneto-encephalographic localization in pediatric epilepsy surgery: comparison with inva-sive intracranial electroencephalography. *Ann Neurol* 1999; **46**: 627–633.

83. Otsubo H, Sharma R, Elliott I, Holowka S, Rutka JT, Snead OC, III Confirmation of two magnetoencephalographic epileptic foci by invasive monitoring from subdural electrodes in an adolescent with right frontocentral epilepsy. *Epilepsia* 1999; **40**: 608–613.

84. Stefan H. Pathophysiology of human epilepsy: imaging and physiologic studies. *Curr Opin Neurol* 2000; **13**: 177–181.

85. Schwartz DP, Badier JM, Vignal JP, Toulouse P, Scarabin JM, Chauvel P. Non-supervised spatio-temporal analysis of interictal magnetic spikes: comparison with intracerebral recordings. *Clin Neurophysiol* 2003; **114**: 438–449.

86. Stefan H, Nimsky C, Scheler G, *et al.* Periventricular nodular heterotopia: A chal-lenge for epilepsy surgery. *Seizure* 2007; **16**: 81–86.

87. Harvey AS, Cross JH, Shinnar S, *et al.* Defining the spectrum of international practice in pediatric epilepsy surgery patients. *Epilepsia* 2008; **49**(1): 146–155.

88. Cross JH, Jayakar P, Nordli D, *et al.* Proposed criteria for referral and evalu-ation of children for epilepsy surgery: recommendations of the subcommission for pediatric epilepsy surgery. *Epilepsia* 2006; **47**: 952–959.

89. Berkovic SF, McIntosh AM, Kalnins RM, *et al.* Preoperative MRI predicts outcome of temporal lobectomy: an actuarial analysis. *Neurology* 1995; **45**: 1358–1363.

90. Chapman K, Wyllie E, Najm I, *et al.* Seizure outcome after epilepsy surgery in patients with normal preoperative MRI. *J Neurol Neurosurg Psychiatry* 2005; **76**: 710–713.

91. RamachandranNair R, Otsubo H, Shroff MM, *et al.* MEG predicts outcome fol-lowing surgery for intractable epilepsy in children with normal or nonfocal MRI findings. *Epilepsia* 2007; **48**: 149–157.

92. Paolicchi JM, Jayakar P, Dean P, *et al.* Predictors of outcome in pediatric epilepsy surgery. *Neurology* 2000; **54**: 642–647.

93. Lee SK, Lee SY, Kim KK, Hong KS, Lee DS, Chung CK. Surgical outcome and prognostic factors of cryptogenic neocortical epilepsy. *Ann Neurol* 2005; **58**: 525–532.

94. Iida K, Otsubo H, Matsumoto Y, *et al.* Characterizing magnetic spike sources by using magnetoencephalography-guided neuronavigation in epilepsy surgery in pediatric patients. *J Neurosurg* 2005; **102**: 187–196.

95. Holowka SA, Otsubo H, Iida K, *et al.* Three-dimensionally reconstructed mag-netic source imaging and neuronavigation in pediatric epilepsy: technical note. *Neurosurgery* 2004; **55**: 1226.

96. Cukiert A, Burattini JA, Mariani PP, *et al.* Extended, one-stage callosal section for treatment of refractory secondarily generalized epilepsy in patients with Lennox–Gastaut and Lennox-like syndromes. *Epilepsia* 2006, **47**: 371–374.

97. Rathore C, Abraham M, Rao RM, *et al.* Outcome after corpus callosotomy in children with injurious drop attacks and severe mental retardation. *Brain and Devel* 2007; **29**: 577–585.

98. Devinski O, Laff R. Callosal lesions and behavior: history and modern concepts. *Epil & Behav*, 2003; **4**: 607–617.

99. Salayev KA, Nakasato N, Ishitobi M, *et al.* Evaluation of interhemispheric time difference by magnetoencephalography before and after total callosotomy. *Neurol Med Chir* (Tokyo) 2006; **46**: 136–142.

100. Mohamed IS, Otsubo H, Donner E, *et al.* Magnetoencephalography for surgical treatment of refractory status epilepticus. *Acta Neurol Scand* 2007; **115** (Suppl 4): 29–36.

Evoked magnetic fields

Contributors

P. G. Simos

A. C. Papanicolaou

E. M. Castillo

D. S. Buchanan

19

Recording evoked magnetic fields (EMFs)

Overview

The capacity to identify relatively small cortical patches that show transient increases in neurophysiological activity (i.e., signaling between neuronal populations) renders MEG suitable for a variety of clinical applications that target stimulus-evoked activity, either during passive stimulation conditions or while the patient is performing a cognitive or linguistic task.

The main purpose of the latter studies is to determine the location and extent of cortex that mediates visual, auditory, somatosensory, motor, and language functions relative to brain regions that need to be surgically removed (e.g., epileptogenic zones or tumors). The goal of these procedures is to reduce the morbidity (i.e., postoperative deficits) that may result if cortical regions containing indispensable components of the brain mechanism for a particular function are compromised during surgery.

A brain mechanism is defined by a set of events that take place in particular brain areas in a particular order and result in the generation of the phenomena, either behavioral or psychological (e.g., perceptual responses), that define each function. When the mechanism is operating, a particular pattern of activation occurs, but this pattern may be difficult to see because it is embedded in the global profile of baseline activity. To isolate the activation pattern for a particular function, a laboratory situation must be contrived to elicit the naturally occurring function on demand, while the participant's brain activity – and activation pattern – is recorded. Stimuli of the same kind as those that naturally trigger the function are presented to the patient. In MEG the magnetic activity at several locations over the head surface is sampled at regular time intervals – potentially temporally contiguous – resulting in a set of time series in response to each external stimulus, a single-trial evoked magnetic field (EMF). When the referral question only requires determination of the location of primary sensory cortex (auditory, visual, or somatosensory), the stimuli are not symbolic (e.g., they may consist of tones, light flashes or geometric patterns, or skin tapping) and the patient may not be asked to process them in a particular manner. When, in contrast, the referral question involves identifying the crucial components of the brain mechanism of language, more complex verbal stimuli are presented in the context of an experimental *task*, and participants are asked to make an overt response (e.g., by pressing a button or by speaking out loud) to indicate that they have processed each stimulus linguistically.

EMFs, much like event-related potentials (ERPs), are waveforms that represent variations of brain activity over time following the onset of an external stimulus. Recent advances in the electronics and software used to reduce the contribution of extraneous sources of magnetic flux to the MEG data have made it possible to detect changes in magnetic flux associated with the presentation of a single stimulus, such as a printed word. Additional procedures are often used, however, to extract activation patterns specific to particular brain functions that are embedded in the global, baseline-activity profile. In the case of MEG, such extraction is accomplished through averaging, which is helpful when the amount of neural signaling for a particular function that differs from baseline is very small.

The early portion of the EMF corresponds to activation of the sensory cortex specific to each type of stimulus (i.e., visual, auditory, or somatic), enabling researchers to identify the brain region responsible for simple sensory functions. In contrast, late portions of the EMF reflect activation of the association cortex. When late activation is mapped, the brain circuits that support higher cognitive functions can be studied in real time, *as* the stimulus is processed and *before* a response is made by the participant.

General instructions for recording EMFs

Stimulation techniques, recording parameters, and general testing conditions in MEG activation studies are very similar to those used in ERP studies. Differences between the two methods arise mainly from the higher susceptibility of MEG to electromagnetic artifacts. The selection of devices used to present stimuli and record the patient's responses must take into account this feature. For instance, many centers prefer mechanical over electrical activation of peripheral nerves. Further, the source of visual or auditory stimuli is located outside of the magnetically shielded chamber, and special stimulus-delivery apparatus are used to transfer light and sound to the patient. In addition to the physical quality of the EMF records, reliable localization of recorded magnetic fields requires a sufficient level of cognitive engagement of the patient in the activation task and, in all cases, that the patient's head remains motionless during each recording session. The duration of these sessions is typically kept short (8 to 10 minutes or less) to ensure optimal compliance.

Replications

Event-related response measurements should be repeated at least twice to establish reproducibility. When stimuli are simple and the goal of the study is to identify the anatomic location of primary sensory cortices, the same set of stimuli may be repeated twice for each receptive area (e.g., finger, ear, or visual hemifield). When the goal of the study is to map the anatomical areas involved in more complex functions, equivalent sets of stimuli (e.g., spoken or printed words) should be developed to prevent familiarization effects. Reproducibility of MEG data is assessed primarily by the stability of estimated source locations of EMF components rather than by the similarity of EMF waveforms, as in the case of ERPs.

Data storage

In addition to online signal averaging, the original waveforms may be stored for off-line analysis, for checking response changes over time, or for eliminating noise-contaminated data before averaging single epochs.

Artifact removal

A number of methods are currently available for removing artifacts. These methods serve two purposes: to remove the artifact and to retain as much information as possible about the signal of interest. If the artifact is rare and has a large amplitude (e.g., eye movement-related artifact), it should be eliminated from the signal. Rare, large amplitude events are very unlikely to average out. At the same time, as many trials as possible should be included in the calculation of the average response, so that one can have the advantage of signal averaging for all of the low-amplitude noise. While the prevention of artifacts during data collection is a priority, many artifacts cannot be eliminated entirely.

The most unrefined – and yet the most direct and reliable – method for eliminating artifacts (i.e., a method that guarantees that the artifact will be removed without removing the signal of interest from the average) is to eliminate any trials that contain artifacts. If one can collect more trials than are needed to obtain good quality averaged responses, one can eliminate artifacts using either automated or manual methods. For instance, by eliminating any events that exceed 75 μV in an auxiliary electro-oculogram (EOG) channel, one can reject eye-blink artifacts. Additionally, criteria can be included for the channel that contains eye artifacts so that only blinks within a certain time range of

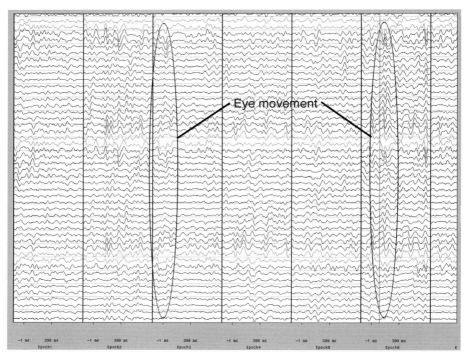

Fig. 19.1. Single-trial EMF epochs containing eye-movement artifacts (EM) which should not be included in the averaging (upper panel). Diffuse noisy epochs, typical of many patient studies, are displayed in the lower panel (opposite). Epochs like these are inadvertently included in further analyses. Unpublished data obtained with a 248-channel axial gradiometer system (Magnes 3600, 4-D Neuroimaging).

the stimulus trigger are eliminated (eye blinks outside the analysis window are not a problem). Examples of ocular artifacts in MEG epochs are shown in Fig. 19.1. This approach can also be used for large movement artifacts that sometimes occur (e.g., during coughing or shifting position). Often, large movement artifacts are selected out by setting an upper bound on the magnetic field strength (~2000 fT) and eliminating any trials that exceed that value in at least one channel.

Visually examining off-line the entire set of waveforms recorded during each session is often useful. Similar to reading EEG waveforms, one should note the presence or absence of abnormalities in background activity, including the dominant rhythm in the occipital region and paroxysmal events such as magnetic spikes, sharp waves, and slow waves. This approach is useful when processing data for auditory and visual evoked fields (EFs), including early sensory

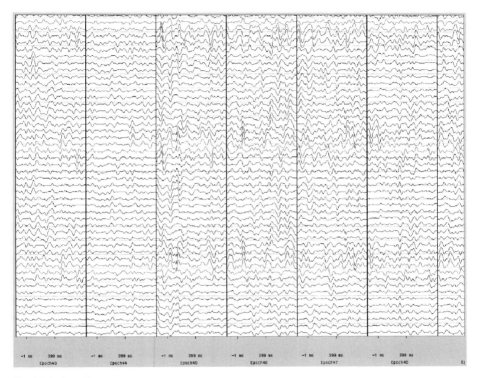

Fig. 19.1. (*cont.*)

components and late components reflecting language-related neurophysiological activation, and for motor mapping.

Removing "bad" channels

If a channel is exceptionally noisy throughout the entire recording session, the recommendation is to not use that channel – to turn it off – for the rest of the analysis. Choosing the bad channels to remove depends on the cause – either technical or physiological – of the noise. If the channel is bad because of technical difficulties with the SQUID, the noise is clearly not physiological and usually has multiple square-wave-type deflections throughout the recording. These channels should be eliminated since they do not provide any useful information regarding brain activity and can dramatically bias source-modeling approaches.

If the channel is bad because of physiological noise, the first approach is to try the previously described artifact-removal options. Sometimes eye blinks can be found throughout the entire data set. If the usual artifact-removal options do not solve the problem, deleting a selected number of channels that are substantially affected by eye blinks can be useful. This is done, for example, if one is not interested in activity from brain areas near the eyes. Most, if not all, MEG analysis programs allow one to toggle bad channels on and off, so that the data, instead of being deleted, are simply not used for display and analysis purposes. Again, retaining as much information as possible, while eliminating as much noise from the signal as possible, should be the goal.

Filtering and electromagnetic-noise reduction

Recorded waveforms normally contain biological signals irrelevant to the purpose of the study (e.g., heart artifacts), system noise (both electronic and mechanical), and environmental noise (electrically and mechanically induced magnetic fields). To reduce the contribution of these signals in the averaged event-related field (ERF), one filters the averaged and/or single-trial recordings. The choice of filter settings is determined by the frequency of the evoked responses sought in a particular MEG study and the nature and intensity of artifacts that are prominent in a particular recording or MEG system. A notch filter may be used when noise of 50 or 60 Hz is caused by AC power sources and cannot be eliminated during recording.

With the exception of myogenic artifacts, most artifacts appear as low-frequency magnetic field fluctuations. The most common sources of these artifacts are movement of the head and body of the patient, as well as movement of metal-containing objects in the vicinity of the MEG recording room. These low-frequency magnetic field fluctuations do not pose a significant problem for somatosensory mapping studies, because high-pass filter settings, usually at 1 to 2 Hz, are sufficient to effectively reduce these extraneous magnetic fields. These artifacts do pose a significant threat to data fidelity when auditory, visual, or movement-related EMFs are recorded, especially when the goal is to map language-related cortex. In those cases high-pass filter settings cannot exceed 0.1 Hz, so special techniques have been developed to monitor extraneous fields and effectively reduce their contribution to the recorded EMFs.

Noise reduction is an important step that allows minimization of the effect of environmental magnetic artifacts over the recorded signals of interest. Environmental noise is typically measured by a subset of reference coils that are located at a sufficient distance – higher in the dewar – from the primary magnetic sensor array to be insensitive to the brain's magnetic signals, yet sufficiently close to the primary sensors to detect the same environmental noise as the primary sensors detect. Fixed fractions of the signals measured by the reference channels are then subtracted from the signals measured by the sensors to reduce the noise component of the MEG tracing. This process can be carried out at several different stages of data acquisition, such as before the data are digitized (real-time analog noise reduction), after they are digitized but before they are stored in a data file (real-time digital noise reduction), and at any time after the data have been acquired (postacquisition noise reduction).

Averaging

Signal averaging remains the norm for extracting signals representing stimulus or task-specific activation from baseline brain activity in MEG studies. Signal averaging requires a trigger that marks the beginning of individual epochs to be averaged. As described above, these triggers can either be generated by a program that delivers stimuli to the subject or by a device that measures when the stimulus is presented to the subject (e.g., a photodiode). After reducing noise-related magnetic fields from individual trials – by filtering, application of special noise-reduction algorithms, single-trial and channel removal – the trials for any one condition are then averaged together. This allows for an increase in SNR by a factor approximately equal to $\sqrt{N}$, where N is the number of trials or single epochs. This relationship is exact when the background noise conforms to a truly Gaussian distribution (white noise), but the relation is only approximate in cases where the noise is not truly random, as is the case with actual brain background activity. Therefore, when a consistent noise source is time-locked to the stimulus, the noise signal will not average out, as is the case with stimulus artifacts from the stimulation device. With the exception of somatosensory studies that require over 250 single epochs at the very least to obtain a usable averaged EMF, the generally accepted number of epochs that are needed to obtain a good SNR is between 100 and 150 trials per condition. This number may be larger or smaller, depending on the amplitude of the signal of interest and the level of background noise.

To be valid, the averaging procedure is subject to a number of assumptions that are unavoidable in all functional-mapping applications of MEG/MSI. The most important assumption is that the signal of interest is exactly time-locked to the stimulus and invariable across trials. If this assumption is not true, the magnetic fields representing neurophysiological activation time-locked to individual stimuli may not be represented in the averaged signal with adequate fidelity.

20

Somatosensory evoked fields (SEFs)

Overview of SEFs

SEFs have been used since the early 1990s to map functionally intact somatosensory cortex [1–6]. Elicited by electrical stimulation of the peripheral nerves or mechanical stimulation of the skin of the upper and lower extremities, body trunk, or head, SEFs have various advantages over somatosensory evoked potentials (SEPs), which are evoked in a similar manner. In particular, the initial components of SEFs (early- and middle-latency peaks) cannot only identify the central sulcus, but also precisely demonstrate the somatotopic organization of the primary sensory cortex [7–10]. In contrast to SEPs, SEFs are particularly useful for functional localization and evaluation of activation within sulci since, unlike EEG that measures both the tangential and radial currents, MEG is mostly sensitive to current sources tangential to the scalp. The sources of SEF components that are obtained through separate mechanical stimulation of each finger, toe, and the perioral area – usually the corner of the lower lip – and modeled as successive single ECDs originate from the contralateral primary sensory cortex within the central sulcus (mostly area 3b). The accuracy of SEF-based central sulcus location estimates has been repeatedly confirmed through comparisons with intraoperative corticography [9, 11–17]. In addition, functional abnormalities along the ascending somatosensory pathways can be quantitatively evaluated by the latency delay with or without concomitant amplitude attenuation [18, 19].

The sensitivity of MEG/MSI for clinical evaluation of the brain mechanism responsible for somatosensory function is further attested by demonstrations of altered somatotopic maps or even complete displacement of the primary somatosensory areas. These changes or displacements have been seen in space-occupying lesions [20–22], early cerebral insult [23], cortical malformations [24, 25], stroke [26–29] and seizure disorders [30].

Such findings suggest that SEF testing is indicated clinically to localize somatosensory function in patients with either organic or functional brain diseases before surgical interventions. Presurgical somatosensory cortex mapping has been used effectively prior to open skull surgery [21, 22, 30–34], stereotactic [6, 15, 35–44], endovascular [21, 34, 45] or radiosurgical procedures [21, 46–48]. SEFs may also be used to evaluate suspected abnormal conditions in the ascending pathways from the peripheral to the central somatosensory system [18, 49–53].

Recording SEFs

In clinical applications – presurgical mapping – the earliest prominent SEF component is used. This component peaks at approximately 20 ms (milliseconds) following electrical stimulation of the median nerve at the wrist and at 45 ms after electrical stimulation of the posterior tibial nerve at the ankle. The earliest, reliably observed SEF peak following mechanical stimulation of the hand is normally observed at approximately 40 ms and at 60 ms when the toes are stimulated. Occasionally, an earlier peak is detectable following mechanical stimulation (at approximately 20 ms to upper- and 40 ms to lower-extremity stimulation, respectively), but these responses are not elicited consistently enough to be of clinical use [54–56].

Stimulation

Electrical stimulation is performed with bipolar adhesive electrodes placed on the skin over the course of the median nerve at the wrist or over the course of the posterior tibial nerve at the ankle (lateral surface). Constant-current pulses with a duration of 0.2 ms are used. Secure grounding of the patient and electrical isolation from the stimulator are important to ensure safety and to minimize stimulation artifacts. Maintaining electrical pulse duration under 0.5 ms serves both patient safety and data quality. Pulse intensity ranges from 5 to 15 mA and is adjusted to the individual threshold that is sufficient to produce twitches of the abductor pollicis brevis muscle, but under the pain threshold. Average stimulation rate is usually 1 or 2 Hz (1 or 2 pulses per second) in order to minimize patient discomfort without greatly prolonging the testing session.

Mechanical stimuli are delivered through an inflatable drum, approximately 1 cm in diameter, clipped to the fingertip or corner of the lower lip with the stimulating piston placed on the glabrous surface of the skin. The drum can be transiently inflated, serving as both a light touch and, primarily, as a pressure stimulus. Typical stimulation parameters for mechanical stimuli are duration, 25 ms; intensity, 2.5 to 3.0 atmospheres (bar), or approximately 15 to 35 pounds per square inch (psi); average stimulation rate, 1.5 to 2.0 Hz. In both normative and patient studies 250 electrical stimuli are sufficient to produce reliable SEFs with acceptable localization results. As with auditory and visual EFs, a slightly variable stimulation rate is employed across stimulus repetitions to reduce habituation effects. When mechanical stimulation is used, up to 500 stimuli may be necessary in order to obtain clinically useful results.

Recording parameters

For clinical applications, SEF segments that sample activity up to 150 ms after stimulus onset and 50 to 100 ms prior to stimulus onset (baseline) are sufficient. The digitization rate is set at a minimum of 640 Hz (samples per second) for mechanical stimulation and 987 Hz for electrical stimulation. High-pass filter settings rarely exceed 1 Hz for mechanical and 10 Hz for electrical stimulation; low-pass filters may be set to a minimum of 40 Hz for mechanical or 150 Hz for electrical. When low-frequency magnetic artifacts are prominent (e.g., in patients with metallic implants), higher high-pass filter settings can be used (2 Hz for mechanical and 10 Hz for electrical stimulation). SEFs can be contaminated by low-frequency noise synchronized with body and head movements in response to stimulation. In this case, fixation of the head and body with padding and adhesive tape may be necessary to minimize the movements. Filter settings may also be adjusted to improve SEF quality (please see below).

Modeling SEF sources as single, successive ECDs by using data from 35 to 37 axial sensors covering the field maxima is sufficient to produce reliable and anatomically plausible source-location estimates. A correlation cutoff between observed and hypothetical SEFs of 0.95 – or goodness of fit greater than 0.90 – is sufficient to ensure reliable location accuracy. In the majority of SEF studies, the best SEF ECDs are associated with a correlation coefficient of 0.98 – and goodness of fit of 0.93 or greater.

Normative SEF data

With mechanical stimulation, first-, second-, and third-digit middle-latency SEFs are obtained more readily and are the most reliable for clinical purposes; however, considerable variability across patients can be present, depending on the location of a perirolandic lesion with respect to the somatotopic hand representation (see Fig. 20.1). Electrical [57] or tactile stimulation, delivered with a wider pneumatic drum than the one used for fingertip stimulation, elicits reliable SEFs in response to stimulation of the skin corresponding to specific dermatomes. Peak latencies of the middle component in response to tactile stimulation corresponding to the cervical (C4), thoracic (Th7), lumbar (L3), and sacral (S1) dermatomes are noted at 26, 36, 49, and 61 ms, respectively [58] (see Fig. 20.2).

Hemispheric asymmetries in the latency of the N20m and P30m peaks are negligible (< 2 ms). Whereas the N20m latency is not affected by stimulus

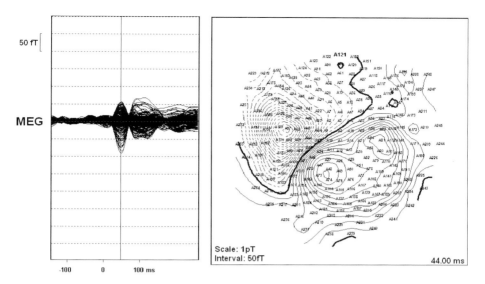

Fig. 20.1. Example of a typical averaged SEF elicited by mechanical stimulation of the index finger. The cursor marks the peak of the middle-latency component peaking at 44 ms. The contour map displays the distribution of magnetic flux at the head surface at the peak of the middle-latency component. Recordings were performed with a 248-channel axial gradiometer system (Magnes 3600, 4-D Neuroimaging).

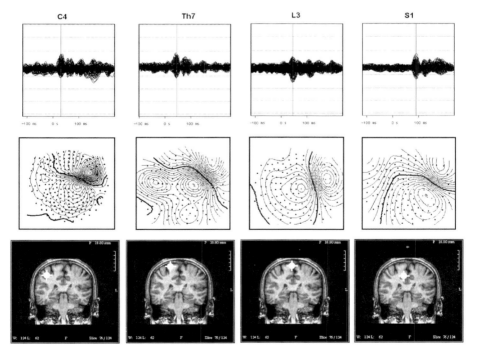

Fig. 20.2. Examples of dermatomal SEFs recorded from a healthy adult participant. Adapted from Castillo & Papanicolaou [58].

Table 20.1. *Normative data for clinically useful SEF peaks*

	Electrical stimulation			
Range (Mean±SD)	Median n: N20m	Median n: P30m	Post. Tibial n. P40m	Trigeminal n.
Latency (young adults) < 4yrs[b]	(20.5 ± 1.5[a]) 17–25 (21 ± 0.5)	32.5 ± 2.6 16–22 (19 ± 0.6)	37–50 (44 ± 6)	21 ± 2[e]
Moment (nA m) (young adults) < 4 yrs	25 ± 10/16 ± 2 2–15 (5 ± 0.6)	30 ± 15/37 ± 3 3–9 (4.7 ± 0.6)	—	—
	Mechanical stimulation			
	Fingertips: N20m	Fingertips	Toes	Lower Lip
Latency	25 ± 2[d]	38–50(42 ± 4)	57 ± 1[c]	24–32 (28 ± 2)
Moment (nA m)	10–30	10–30	–	10–30

The data reported here have been pooled from several studies using a variety of recording devices ranging from 28 to 306 channel systems. SD = standard deviation; nA m = nanoAmpere meters; n = nerve; post. = posterior; yrs = years.
[a] May be slightly delayed in the elderly (a mean of 24 ms reported by Stephen [63]). In healthy neonates the equivalents of the N20m and P30m peaks occur at approx. 30 and 60 ms, respectively [64]. The most readily detectable response in neonates to mechanical stimulation is at 64 ± 12 ms (with a product moment of 9 ± 5 nA m [64]).
[b] [60].
[c] [65].
[d] Not reliably obtained.
[e] Electrical stimulation of the lower lip [66].

intensity (above the sensory threshold) or stimulus repetition rate (between 1 and 4 Hz), P30m latency is significantly reduced with increasing intensity and stimulation rate. The field magnitude of both components increases with stimulus intensity [59], although the ratio of P30m to N20m amplitude is consistently over 2:1. Normative SEF data compiled from several published studies are presented in Table 20.1.

SEFs can be reliably recorded under anesthesia for patients who are unable to cooperate (i.e., unable to remain motionless during the recording sessions). Anesthesia is typically induced with intravenous administration of propofol, which can be titrated to the lowest dose necessary to keep the patient still. This procedure is especially useful for presurgical referrals of infants and young children. In a recently reported patient series, SEFs were obtained under sedation to (electrical) median nerve stimulation and reliably localized in 79% of hemispheres studied [60]. The early SEF peaks from electrical stimulation of the median nerve show minimal effects of sleep stage [61].

Sleep stage has more profound effects on SEF waveform morphology in neonates. The earliest SEF deflection is best obtained during quiet sleep and has a widely variable peak latency, ranging from 100 to approximately 200 ms [62].

The anatomical location of neurophysiological activation that gives rise to the recorded SEFs is estimated, in essentially all clinical applications, using the single ECD model. The algorithm is applied to data recorded from a small set of sensors (typically 35 to 37) centered at the reversal point of the field pattern indicative of the presence of a dipolar source – in the case of magnetometer or axial gradiometer sensors – or at the field maximum – in the case of planar gradiometer systems. ECD solutions are obtained for a few successive data points around the peak of the component of interest and spanning 10 to 15 ms around this peak. The best ECD solution based on correlation or goodness of fit is then chosen to represent the sources responsible for the generation of each component.

The most reliably elicited components across patients are the early responses (N20m and P40m for median and posterior tibial nerve stimulation, respectively) and the middle-latency responses to mechanical stimulation (peaking at approximately 40 ms for fingertips, 60 ms for toes, and 17 ms for the lower lip). The test–retest stability of source-localization parameters is greater for first- than for fifth-digit stimulation [67] and was estimated in normal subjects to be in the order of 4 and 8 mm (millimeters), respectively. In patients, test–retest stability estimates are slightly worse in the affected hemisphere, ranging between 1.6 and 19 mm (geometric distance), 0 to 2.6 ms for the N20m latency, and 0.9 to 23 fT for N20m field strength [68], using mechanical stimulation. In general the yield, defined as the proportion of patients with reliably localizable SEFs, is similar for electrical and tactile stimulation of the upper limbs but favors electrical stimulation for the lower limbs.

Aberrant SEFs

Atypical SEFs, ranging from aberrant amplitude and/or latency of one or more of the prominent SEF components to unusual forms of the cortical somatosensory maps, have been reported in a variety of neurological conditions. While examples of such findings are presented below, solid clinical applications have not yet been derived from them. For instance, the amplitude of middle-latency SEFs (mechanical stimulation) is often larger in the hemisphere that contains a mass lesion than in the nonaffected hemisphere [69]. This difference was found for tumors near the somatosensory cortex, which were nevertheless not associated with significant displacement of the SEF sources, and not for tumors in more remote areas.

Enhanced amplitude of middle-latency electrically elicited SEFs (P30m and N60m) has also been reported in some patients with rolandic epilepsy. Peak latency and amplitude of the earlier N20m peak are typically not affected; this finding probably reflects a state of hyperexcitability of the primary and secondary somatosensory cortex [70]. In contrast, reduced amplitude and/or delayed latency of the N20m component are common findings following a cerebrovascular accident (CVA) in perirolandic regions, although increased latency of the P30m component (electrical stimulation) has also been seen when compared to the healthy-side SEF [71]).

Aberrant localization of SEF sources has been reported in several studies. In general, atypical somatosensory map layout is more likely found in congenital malformations, such as arterioventricular malformations (AVMs) [24], focal cortical dysplasia, polymicrogyria, and schizencephaly [25]. Deviations from the "normal" pattern may be as dramatic as the presence of a complete ipsilateral representation of the body surface [24]. Atypical maps may also be associated with lesions incurred later in life [20]. Interestingly, the extent of the presumed reorganization of the somatosensory cortex does not always correlate with the severity – or absence thereof – of sensory deficits. Moreover, the amplitude of the N20m component in the acute phase of post-middle-cerebral-artery stroke does not appear to predict the degree of sensorimotor recovery assessed several months after the event [72, 73].

Referral questions that may be addressed with SEFs

The key indication for performing somatosensory mapping with MEG/MSI is determination of the location of the primary somatosensory cortex and its spatial proximity to a mass lesion or epileptogenic zone [30]. This referral question is answered by examining the anatomic location of the sources of the early-latency (electrical stimulation) and middle-latency (tactile stimulation) SEF peaks. Some authors advocate the use of localization information derived not only from the early-latency, but also the middle-latency components [74]. In healthy participants the "best" sources of the N20m and P30m responses are not consistently different across cases, although a tendency for the latter to be found in the precentral gyrus (anterior wall of the central sulcus) in a small proportion of subjects has been reported [59]. Sample SEF data from a patient with a right central cystic lesion are presented in Fig. 20.3.

For MEG/MSI results to have clinical utility, SEF source localizations must accurately indicate the location of cortex indispensable for somatosensory function. This accuracy assumes adequate stability of source parameters – mainly source location – over time. As evidenced by the normative SEF data discussed

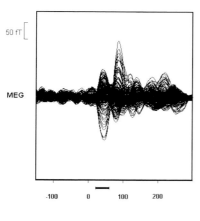
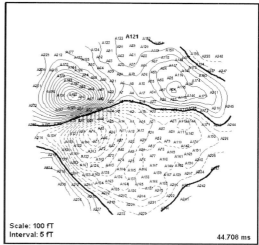

Fig. 20.3. Upper set of images: SEF waveform associated with mechanical stimulation of the right index finger and contour map at the peak of the middle-latency component (peaking at 44 ms) in a patient suffering from a frontal cystic lesion. Lower set of images (overleaf): source locations that best account for the middle-latency components of SEFs elicited by mechanical stimulation of the right index (black square) and middle fingers (white square). Unpublished data, MEG Laboratory, University of Texas Health Science Center at Houston.

above, the stability requirement appears to be met. The question of the *concurrent validity* of SEF source-localization data, however, has been addressed mostly indirectly by comparing SEF source locations with estimates of the location of the (primary) somatosensory cortex obtained through preoperative or intraoperative SEP recordings and/or electrical-stimulation mapping. The mean distance between the SEF source location and the location of the somatosensory cortex obtained invasively has been reported to be 1 cm or less in adult tumor patients [17, 75] and pediatric epilepsy patients [76].

A clinical question far more important than concurrent validity is *predictive validity* – whether SEF mapping results help to improve surgical outcome. Predictive validity of somatosensory MEG/MSI mapping, however, is not as easy to assess. This assessment would require data on the relation between proximity of the SEF sources to the borders of the lesion and clinical outcome. Studies addressing this issue thus far have not provided a conclusive answer, mainly because decisions for the optimal surgical approach usually take into account the results of the MEG/MSI study for referred patients. As a result of this practice, a control group of patients having surgery without MEG-derived localization results is not available in reported patient series.

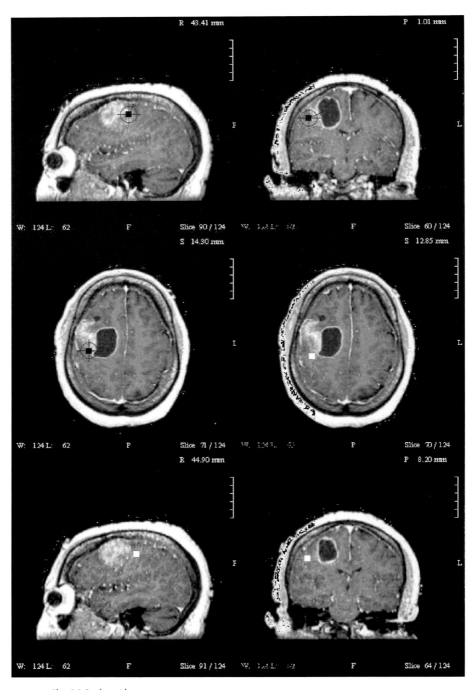

Fig. 20.3. (cont.)

Results from relatively large patient series published thus far can be summarized as follows. One study reported that 45% of 119 patients with gliomas who were evaluated with MEG/MSI were deemed suitable for surgery (based on postoperative functional risk assessment) and only 6% experienced neurological deterioration [33]. This figure compared favorably with functionally significant or permanent deficits in 17% to 20% of the operated patients reported in other studies (e.g., Romstock and coworkers [77]). In another patient series, tumor resection was performed in 27 patients with a tumor or AVM and preoperative MEG/MSI studies (22 operations were aided by frameless stereotaxy [36]). Of interest in this study were 5 patients with lesion borders located at a distance of 4 mm or less from the SEF sources. Only one of these patients showed a transient motor deficit (weakness) [36].

Firsching and colleagues [42] performed preoperative SEF mapping in 30 patients with tumors around the central sulcus, in 21 of whom "the tumor had direct contact with the sensorimotor cortex, as determined by MEG." MEG/MSI data were taken into account in order to maximize tumor resection while preserving presumed functional cortex. All of the 10 patients without preoperative motor deficits remained deficit free after surgery. Of the remaining 18 patients with preoperative motor deficits, 7 showed symptom improvement at discharge, 10 were unchanged at discharge, and only 1 patient showed persisting postoperative deterioration. In an even larger patient series with 106 tumor patients – but 3- to 7-day postoperative functional-assessment data were available in only 48 – SEF sources were found in tumor tissue in 16% of the patients and immediately adjacent to the tumor margin in 8% of the patients [78]. Patients who underwent partial resection to preserve tissue in which SEF sources were previously found tended to show less postoperative deficit (of the 14 patients with partial resection, 9 were unchanged or improved and 5 were worse), but the tendency was not statistically significant. However, in 9 of 11 patients with SEF sources in normal tissue who underwent total resection, function was preserved, whereas in the 2 patients with SEF sources sited within the tumor, function worsened after total resection. Only recently has SEF mapping been used for planning stereotactic irradiation treatment with promising results [48].

A relatively safe conclusion to be drawn from these studies is that the distance between SEF sources and borders of a mass lesion is strongly correlated to the risk of postoperative sensory and/or motor deficits. However, the localization accuracy of MEG for the primary somatosensory area may be affected by scar tissue and/or skull deformities due to prior surgery in the same region. These factors may also affect the accuracy of intraoperative corticography. The use of frameless stereotactic systems may help improve the accuracy of coregistration of MEG sources on the exposed brain during surgery and may, therefore, improve the degree of concordance between MEG and intraoperative corticography (see, for instance, Schulder and colleagues [79]).

21

Movement-related magnetic fields (MRFs) – motor evoked fields (MEFs)

Overview of MRFs

Magnetic fields preceding voluntary movements are generated by neurons oriented tangential to the scalp in motor cortex contralateral to the limb moved. MRFs can be recorded and their intracranial sources localized with much greater fidelity and reliability than movement-related potentials [80–87]. The location of MRF sources in the anterior wall of the central sulcus has been confirmed in several studies through direct comparisons with the results of direct electrocortical-stimulation mapping [32, 36, 75].

MRFs are used clinically to localize the central sulcus and the somatotopic organization of the primary motor cortex or to evaluate motor function in patients with either organic or functional brain diseases before surgical interventions such as craniotomy [22], stereotactic [15, 36, 37, 40, 43], or radiosurgical procedures [88], and/or with suspected abnormalities in the descending corticospinal pathways [70].

Recording MRFs

Elicitation

Extension of the index finger is most commonly used for eliciting MRFs. Extension of the entire hand may also be used. Movement can be self-paced or externally cued. During a self-paced recording session, the patient lies supine, hand at his/her side resting on a nonmagnetic pad, and is asked to briskly flex the index finger at a rate of approximately one movement every 3 to 5 seconds (see Fig. 21.1). In the context of externally cued procedures, the patient is asked to react by pushing a button or performing hand extension as quickly as possible to a visual [36] or tactile [32] cue that is presented every 2 to 3 seconds. At most centers, somatosensory and motor mapping are performed in separate sessions.

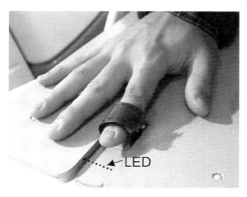

Fig. 21.1. Finger movement pad used to trigger MRFs. When the small plate fixed to the index finger interrupts the light-emitting diode because of finger extension, an input is triggered. From Oishi and coworkers [22], with permission.

Recently, a procedure for mapping both somatosensory and motor functions in the same session has been developed [32]. In this protocol, mechanical tactile stimulation is applied to the subject's index finger and serves as a cue for the individual to perform a full wrist extension.

The clinical yield – percentage of successful MEG studies – of these techniques is reportedly very high, ranging from 80% to 90% across studies. The most frequent reason for failure to obtain reliable MRFs in individual patients is the presence of preoperative motor deficits (hemiparesis or weakness).

Triggering

Onset of hand or finger movement serves as a trigger to temporally align MRF epochs and is marked by the onset of the electromyograph (EMG) peak recorded from the moving hand or by the onset of an electrical pulse generated by a button [36] or by a light diode [22]. When motion rise-time is not consistent among trials due to a motor deficit, larger signals can be obtained by processing the MRFs off-line after visually determining EMG onset from the raw data. Some centers routinely use the EMG peak for aligning MRF epochs [75] (see below).

Recording parameters

Approximately 70 to 100 artifact-free epochs are usually sufficient to obtain reliable MRFs. Epochs include a 500 to 1000 ms premovement and a 200 ms postmovement period. The first 200 ms of the prestimulus period is used to obtain baseline data. A minimum sampling rate of 500 Hz and a band-pass filter set between 0.1 and 40 Hz are sufficient, but if necessary, a high-pass filter setting of 1 Hz can be used. Placement of the helmet-like sensor should ensure coverage of the anterior-lateral region of the skull where MRF maxima are usually recorded. EMGs of the extensor digitorum superficialis and flexor digitorum superficialis muscles are recorded simultaneously.

Eye- and body-movement artifacts

Based on their morphology and scalp distribution, MRFs are more susceptible to ocular artifacts than SEFs. Moreover, the setting of the high-pass filter used to record and process MRFs rarely exceeds 1 Hz, making reduction of the amplitude of movement-related – including ocular – artifacts difficult. Preventing the occurrence of such artifacts in the recorded data is, therefore, essential. To prevent eye movements from synchronizing with motor responses, one can use a visual fixation point. Eye blinking can be reduced during measurement periods by introducing breaks in recording. In addition, the body and head are immobilized to prevent their synchronous movement with the target limb. A cushion under the target limb will prevent vibration from occurring when the limb returns to its original position at the end of the movement.

Normative MRF data

The component of the MRF used to obtain estimates of motor cortex location varies considerably across centers and across patients within the same center. Across activation protocols, however, two clinically useful components of the MRF are commonly seen. The earliest peak is noted on average at 30 to 40 ms (ranging from 60 to 0 ms) prior to EMG onset. This magnetic activity arises from the contralateral primary motor cortex and reflects neurophysiological activity closely linked to corticospinal efferent volleys [89]. In activation protocols involving a button press, this component peaks between approximately 45 and 80 ms prior to the patient's response. The second component, larger in amplitude, peaks on average at approximately 100 ms after EMG onset, and presumably reflects motor cortex activation associated with the processing of proprioceptive input from the moving limb. In the context of the mechanically triggered protocol [32], SEF components are noted first, at approximately 40 ms after delivery of the stimulus, followed by activation of the secondary somatosensory cortex, lasting for approximately 200 ms (see Figs. 21.2 and 21.3). Both peaks reportedly provide accurate estimates of motor cortex location, although the clinical yield of the second MRF component is considerably higher [90].

Modeling intracranial sources at the peak of the MRF components as ECDs by using data from 35 to 37 axial sensors covering the field maxima is sufficient to provide reliable estimates of underlying motor cortex activity. A correlation

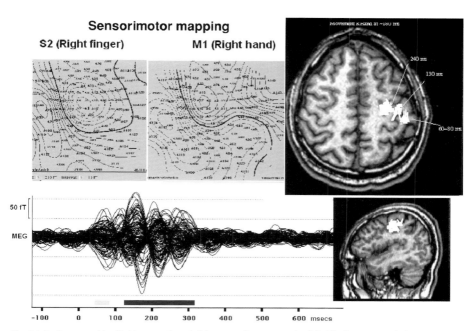

Fig. 21.2. Averaged isofield maps (top left), sensorimotor evoked fields (bottom right) and estimated ECD locations (right-hand portion) as derived from a healthy volunteer. The middle-latency SEF component elicited by the tactile cue is evident first (marked by the light gray bar) followed by a sequence of motor responses preceding and overlapping with the onset of the hand movement (around 160 ms in this case, dark gray bar). Estimated ECDs representing activity in the primary somatosensory (triangles) and motor cortices (squares) are displayed on the sagittal image of the participant's MRI. Adapted from Castillo and coworkers [32].

cutoff between observed and hypothetical MRFs of 0.95 – or goodness of fit of 0.90 or more – is sufficient to ensure acceptable levels of localization accuracy.

While test–retest stability data for MRFs are scarce (e.g., see Rosburg and associates [91]), concurrent validity estimates are generally comparable to those of SEFs. On average, the distance between the location of the "best" MRF ECD and the estimated location of primary motor cortex using invasive procedures is in the order of 10 mm. The latter is defined as the site associated with maximum EMG activity elicited by direct cortical stimulation or the site of polarity reversal of the somatosensory evoked response elicited by median-nerve stimulation and recorded intraoperatively [17, 75].

Common findings in patients with perirolandic lesions include attenuated MRFs, which occasionally prevent reliable localization of intracranial sources,

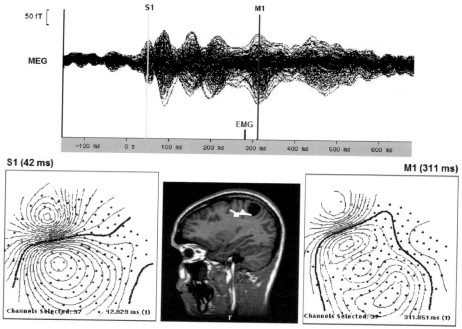

Fig. 21.3. Top: averaged MRF waveforms from the affected hemisphere of a patient with a parietal cystic lesion. The middle-latency SEF component elicited by the tactile cue is present first (S1) followed by the onset of EMG activity in the contralateral hand. Corresponding contour maps at the peaks of the SEF and MRF components are shown in the lower left and lower right portions of the figure. Estimated ECDs representing activity in the primary somatosensory (triangle) and motor (square) cortices are displayed in the sagittal image of the patient's MRI in relation to the lesion. Adapted from Castillo and coworkers [32].

and reduction of the distance between hand (median-nerve or fingertip) SEF sources and early MRF courses [22].

Referral questions that may be addressed with MRFs

The basic referral question addressed with MRFs concerns localization of the primary motor cortex in patients with either mass lesions or suspected epileptogenic zones in perirolandic areas. In many cases SEFs may be sufficient for presurgical planning, especially when the targeted area lies posterior to a clearly demarcated central sulcus (see, for instance, Kirsch and coworkers [92]). In cases, however, when a mass lesion distorts local gyral anatomy to such an extent that identification of the full course of the central sulcus is not possible and/or when the lesion is located near the anterior wall of a (possibly) discernible central sulcus, motor mapping is indicated.

Because of the difficulty in obtaining MRFs time-locked to orofacial or lower limb movement, most clinical applications of MRFs involve mapping the hand motor area. Unfortunately, the predictive validity of MEG/MSI motor mapping performed either alone or in combination with somatosensory mapping has not been assessed systematically; the general impression from reports of large patient series is that motor mapping can provide valuable information in preoperative risk assessment and planning [37].

22

Auditory evoked magnetic fields (AEFs)

Overview of AEFs

AEFs to monaural or binaural stimulation have several advantages over auditory evoked potentials (AEPs) elicited in a similar manner. Unlike AEPs, AEFs can clearly and easily distinguish bilateral responses. Thus, any unilateral abnormality or interhemispheric difference between auditory cortices can be accurately detected [5, 93–95]. In addition, any abnormal auditory function can be quantitatively evaluated by variations in latency with or without amplitude attenuation [96, 97].

AEFs can be used clinically to localize the auditory cortex and to evaluate auditory function in patients with (1) either organic or functional brain diseases before surgical interventions such as craniotomy [39, 96], endovascular, or radiosurgical procedures [98, 99], and/or (2) suspected abnormal conditions in the ascending pathways from the peripheral to the central auditory system [100–106].

Recording AEFs

AEF sources

For most clinical purposes, the M100 component of the AEF is analyzed. This component peaks on average at 90 ms after the onset of the stimulus at the subject's ear (in older children and adults) and corresponds to the vertex-negative N100 response in AEPs. Intracranial sources that account for the peak of the M100 response can be localized reliably in the supratemporal plane in the close vicinity of Heschl's gyrus [107, 108]. However, magnetic activity at and slightly after the M100 peak may be produced by anatomically distinct auditory cortex generators. Evidence from parallel intracerebral and MEG recordings showed that early portions of M100 activity coincide with electrophysiological activity inside Heschl's gyrus, whereas later activity may originate in the planum temporale [109].

Stimulation

When the goal of the MEG/MSI study is localization of the sources of the M100 component, monaural stimulation contralateral to the affected hemisphere is preferable. Tone-burst stimuli of usually 1 kHz frequency, 50 to 200 ms duration, 5 to 10 ms rise-and-fall times, and measuring 80 to 90 decibels (dB) sound pressure level (SPL) at the patient's ear are most commonly used. Stimuli may be produced by a computer sound card and delivered through plastic tubes to ear-inserts. The time delay between the generation of the stimulus and its arrival at the patient's ear depends on the length of the air tube and must be measured in order to estimate actual AEF component latencies (for 3-meter-long tubes the delay is approximately 9 ms). Stimuli are presented with a randomly variable interstimulus interval (ISI) to prevent habituation. A good compromise ensuring sufficiently long ISIs and a recording session not exceeding 3 minutes involves presentation of 100 stimuli at a rate of one stimulus per 1 to 2 seconds. Longer ISIs, averaging approximately 3 seconds, may be needed for younger patients in order to maximize M100 field strength and minimize its peak latency [110].

Recording parameters

Approximately 70 to 100 artifact-free epochs are usually sufficient to obtain reliable AEFs. Epochs may consist of a 100 to 150 ms prestimulus and a 300 ms poststimulus period. A minimum sampling rate of 254 Hz and a band-pass filter set between 0.1 and 40 Hz are sufficient to optimize M100 parameters; but, if necessary, a high-pass filter setting of 1 Hz can be used. As in the case of MRFs, AEF morphology and scalp distribution renders them susceptible to ocular artifacts. Moreover, the high-pass filter setting used to record and process AEFs rarely exceeds 1 Hz, making reduction of the amplitude of movement-related – including ocular – artifacts difficult. Preventing the occurrence of these movement-related artifacts in the recorded data is, therefore, essential.

The M100 component of the AEF is greatly affected by the level of alertness of the patient. Before testing, one should confirm that the patient had an adequate amount of sleep on the previous night, as the state of wakefulness is critical for the study. The occipital alpha rhythm in the ongoing MEG can be used to monitor wakefulness. During the study, the patient should be instructed to maintain eye fixation to reduce ocular artifacts and the occurrence of prominent alpha waves. However, the patient need not perform specific tasks that require manual responses or counting stimuli.

Normative AEF data

Latency of the M100 component is shorter and amplitude is larger in the hemisphere contralateral to the stimulated ear than in the hemisphere ipsilateral to stimulation [5, 108, 111]. On average, this difference is in the order of 10 ms. M100 peak latencies tend to be slightly shorter and amplitudes larger in the right hemisphere than in the left, regardless of the side of stimulus delivery [93]. On average, tone-elicited M100 peaks in healthy adults are noted at 90 ($\pm$9) ms for contralateral and at 100 ($\pm$9) ms for ipsilateral stimulation. Latencies are longer in older children by 10 to 20 ms [110]. Field strength varies widely across participants, with the majority of cases ranging from 50 to 100 fT. Among full-term, healthy infants younger than 6 months, AEF morphology differs dramatically [112, 113]. In some infants the AEF is dominated by a single deflection peaking at 250 ms and a peak latency decreasing with age to approximately 150 ms at 6 months. In other infants two peaks (at approximately 150 and 350 ms) occur. Use of an oddball procedure may help improve fidelity of AEF peaks in this age group [112].

Modeling M100 sources as single, successive ECDs by using data from 35 to 40 sensors covering the field maxima is sufficient to produce reliable and anatomically plausible source-location estimates, at least in adult participants. A correlation cutoff between observed and hypothetical AEFs of 0.95 – or goodness of fit 0.90 or more – is sufficient to ensure reliable location accuracy. In young children, source localizations are less reliable, and this may be due in part to the inadequacy of the single ECD model to take into account magnetic flux originating from the opposite – ipsilateral to the stimulating ear – hemisphere [114]. Unfortunately no alternative or better localization technique is currently available for those cases. ECD moment also varies considerably across participants, ranging in most cases between 10 and 30 nA m. Interhemispheric asymmetries in source location are commonly noted, with more anterior M100 peak source locations in the right than in the left hemisphere [5, 115], a finding that may be related to hemispheric differences in the spatial layout of the Sylvian fissure.

The test–retest reliability of M100 parameters is reportedly very good. Using a planar gradiometer system and tone stimuli in the context of an oddball task with adult participants, Virtanen and colleagues [116] reported two-day test–retest variability in M100 latency averaging 2 to 3 ms, 20% of the total field strength, and best ECD moment. Mean linear ECD distance between measurements obtained on different days was 2 mm.

Aberrant AEFs

Patients with structural brain lesions also show changes in AEFs. Mäkelä and coworkers reported that the N100m on the affected side was absent in patients with large ischemic lesions near the auditory cortex and that the N100m latency was prolonged in patients with ischemic lesions in the frontal lobe [98, 117]. Nakasato and colleagues reported that the M100 showed prolonged latency or was absent in patients with brain tumors near the auditory cortex and that the abnormal latency could become normalized after tumor surgery [96]. M100 peak latencies of up to 123 ms were found in some cases. A similar delay in peak M100 latency was found in patients with epileptic spikes arising from the superior temporal lobe in the absence of structural lesions [118]. Mizuno and associates [119] reported that the ECD strength of the N100m in the affected hemisphere was smaller than in the normal hemisphere in patients with corticobasal degeneration, possibly caused by a neuronal loss in the primary auditory cortex. Normal asymmetry of the N100m of the AEFs is preserved in patients with atypical, right hemispheric language dominance [94].

Aberrant AEFs have also been reported in dyslexia, schizophrenia, and autism. For instance, the difference in M100 peak amplitude in the left hemisphere, between speech and nonspeech analogous stimuli, is reportedly reduced in adults with a history of dyslexia as compared to nonimpaired readers [120]. Another study reported that the expected asymmetry in the location of the cortical source of the M100 response – more anterior in the right compared to the left hemisphere – was observed in the control group but not in a group of children with reading impairment [121].

Two recent studies have focused on the characteristics of the M100 response elicited by tone stimuli in children and adolescents with autism. Gage and colleagues [122] reported that the dynamic range of M100 modulation – the difference between the M100 latency at the lowest frequency and the M100 latency at the highest frequency tested – was significantly smaller in the right and greater in the left hemisphere for the group of children with autism compared to the age-matched controls. More recently, Oram Cardy and coworkers [123] used a two-tone procedure and reported the reduced probability for detecting the M100 component in response to the second tone among children and adolescents with autism compared to typically developing children. However, these promising demonstrations have yet to give rise to useful clinical applications.

Referral questions that may be addressed with AEFs

The most common application of AEFs is presurgical planning in cases of lesions encroaching on the auditory cortex. In those cases, however, language mapping should also be performed to help determine hemispheric dominance for language. Tone AEFs can then be used to identify the location of the primary auditory cortex with higher accuracy than that afforded by the early components (M100) of language-related fields.

23

Visual evoked magnetic fields (VEFs)

Overview of VEFs

Mapping the precise location of the primary visual cortex may be indicated prior to resecting mass lesions in the vicinity of the calcarine fissure. VEFs evoked by monocular or binocular stimulation have various advantages in comparison with the visual evoked potentials (VEPs) elicited in a similar manner. Unlike VEPs, VEFs clearly and easily distinguish bilateral occipital responses from each other using left- or right-hemifield stimuli [124–127]. A unilateral abnormality in the visual cortex or interhemispheric difference between the left and right cortices can, therefore, be easily and accurately detected. The intracranial sources that give rise to the early component of the magnetic waveform evoked by rapidly changing patterned stimulation are used as markers of the primary visual area [124, 128–132]. Hemifield or single-quadrant stimulation has been used successfully to localize visual cortex in patients with organic brain diseases before surgical interventions involving craniectomy [33, 39] and stereotactic procedures [133]. In addition, any abnormal visual function can be quantitatively evaluated by the latency delay with or without amplitude attenuation [99, 134].

Recording VEFs

VEF sources

In VEFs evoked by pattern-reversal stimulation, the responses with latency shorter than 200 ms are considered to arise from the primary visual cortex. The sources of the P100m response that peaks at approximately 100 ms after stimulus onset, which corresponds to the P100 VEP response, is typically studied in clinical settings.

Stimulation

In a typical recording session, stimuli consist of half-field checkerboard patterns subtending 30 degrees of visual angle, changing every 1 sec (second) to introduce a complete local brightness reversal while maintaining a constant average luminance. A trigger is generated every time a reversal takes place. Approximately 200 such reversals are presented.

For clinical purposes, visual stimulus-delivery systems consist of an LCD projector located immediately outside the magnetically shielded chamber that projects through a series of mirrors to a back-projection screen situated in the patient's line of vision. For patients with myopia, visual acuity should be corrected with nonmagnetic lenses.

The ability to obtain VEFs with a high degree of fidelity depends in part on the technical characteristics of the projector used. Most generic projectors show significant *variability* in the onset time, i.e., when the projector receives the signal from the stimulus control unit – usually a computer – to when the signal is displayed. If variability is significant, i.e., greater than 5 to 10 ms, a signal from a photosensor should be used as a trigger. When the absolute latency of the VEF responses is of interest, the *delay* of the projector – the time the signal is received until the time the stimulus is presented on the screen – must be determined. Most LCD projectors introduce an approximately 30 ms delay. Two primary types of projectors are currently being used for MEG studies: LCD and DLP (digital light-processing) projectors. Although DLP projectors have the best temporal characteristics for MEG studies – generally low variability (<1 ms) and small onset delay (~3 ms) – the price of these projectors is often prohibitive.

Recording parameters

The typical sampling rate is between 290 to 600 Hz while filters are set between 0.1 and 30 Hz. An epoch duration of 300 to 400 ms including a 100 ms prestimulus interval is sufficient for clinical applications of VEFs. Although contamination of the VEF epochs by ocular artifacts is not particularly problematic due to the location of the field maxima, maintaining eye fixation on the stimulation screen is essential. When the patient cannot fixate well, full-field stimulation may be used. Since having the patient in a state of wakefulness is critical for the study, one must confirm that the patient has had adequate sleep on the night before VEF testing. The occipital alpha rhythm in ongoing spontaneous MEG can be used to monitor wakefulness. The MEG helmet should be placed so that a sufficient number of recording channels is near the occipital region.

Modeling P100m sources as single, successive ECDs by using data from 35 to 40 axial sensors covering the field maxima is sufficient to produce reliable and anatomically plausible source-location estimates, at least in adult participants.

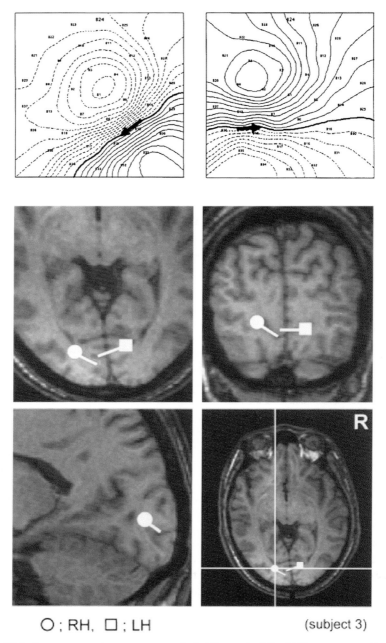

O : RH,   □ : LH   (subject 3)

Fig. 23.1. Upper row: contour maps computed at the peak of the P100m component to left- (left-hand image) and right-hemifield stimulation (right-hand image). Lower set of images: best ECDs accounting for the VEF distributions at 105 ms following stimulus reversal (RH, LH: right- and left-hemifield stimulus, respectively). Reprinted with permission from Nakamura and coworkers [125].

A correlation cutoff between observed and hypothetical AEFs of 0.95 – or goodness of fit 0.90 or more – is sufficient to ensure reliable location accuracy. An example of typical VEF data is presented in Fig. 23.1.

Normative VEF data

The neural origin of the P100 visual response to pattern reversals of half-field stimulation is typically found in the fundus of the calcarine fissure. With the exception of the study by Armstrong and coworkers [135], population norms for MEG/MSI VEFs are not available. On the basis of data from 100 subjects, 18 to 87 years of age, who were tested with a second-order gradiometer system in an unshielded environment, a population latency range of 90 to 120 ms for the P100m component to half-field stimulation was reported.

Aberrant VEFs

Displaced ECD sources or VEFs with prolonged latencies are often found in the affected hemisphere of patients with occipital lesions, with prolonged latency VEFs being more commonly seen [136]. Aberrant VEF morphology has also been reported in various neurological conditions associated with visual system abnormalities [25, 99, 134, 137–141]. Neurophysiological activity that takes place during the advanced stages of print processing – processing words or word-like stimuli – and that is reflected in VEF components observed after the P100m component in visual association cortices and, most importantly, in posterior superior temporal, temporoparietal, and frontal regions, has been extensively studied in an effort to identify aberrant patterns of cortical engagement associated with developmental reading disability (dyslexia). Although reading studies are not part of routine clinical protocols, the robustness of these findings is worth exploring further and will be reviewed briefly in Chapter 24. Unfortunately, the sensitivity or predictive value of VEFs is not definitively better than that of the cheaper and easier to obtain visual evoked responses (VERs) to be of clinical use for purposes other than presurgical mapping.

Referral questions that may be addressed with VEFs

VEFs can be indicated clinically to localize visual cortex in patients with organic brain diseases before surgical interventions, such as craniotomy [33, 39] (see Fig. 23.2), stereotactic [133], or radiosurgical procedures [48]. However, presurgical mapping using VEFs is not requested as often as somatosensory, motor, or language mapping, in part due to the low relative incidence of mass lesions or

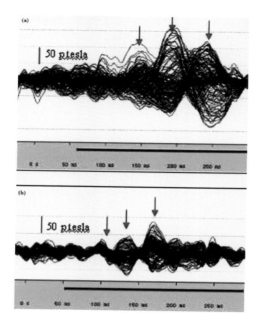

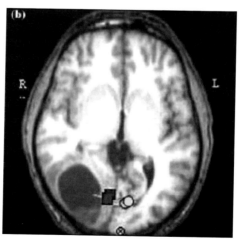

Fig. 23.2. VEFs recorded from a patient with a right occipital cystic lesion from the affected (upper set of waveforms, left-hemifield stimulation) and the unaffected hemisphere (lower set of waveforms, right-hemifield stimulation). Notice the significant delay in the peak latency of the P100m component in the affected side compared to the unaffected side (arrows). Lower panel: location of ECDs to left-hemifield (squares) and right-hemifield (circles) stimulation in relation to the lesion. Adapted with permission from Grover and coworkers [136].

epileptogenic zones in the occipital cortex. The largest patient series reported thus far included 18 patients with usable data [136]. Only 1 of 13 patients who presented with preoperative visual deficits did not produce VEF responses in the affected hemisphere. The authors concluded that VEFs, when indicated, can be very useful in planning the surgical approach and determining the extent of the resection.

24

Language-related brain magnetic fields (LRFs)

Overview of LRFs

When language stimuli are presented acoustically or visually, not only is neurophysiological activation elicited in the primary auditory and visual cortices, but also in a number of areas of the brain responsible for language functions. The characteristics of this activation depends to a certain extent upon the task that the patient is asked to perform on these stimuli, typically appearing as late language-related brain magnetic fields (LRFs) after the primary sensory components [115, 142]. These late components localize to language-related areas of the brain regardless of the modality of stimulus presentation [142]. LRFs are repeatable [142–144] and have been validated by comparison with the Wada procedure [75, 143, 145–149] and electrocortical stimulation mapping [142, 150, 151]. Most LRF studies have focused on receptive language areas, although frontal expressive language [148, 152] and basal temporal areas [153] have been studied as well.

Recordings of LRFs are indicated clinically to (1) determine the language-dominant hemisphere and (2) identify cortex indispensable for language functions in patients with either organic or functional brain diseases before surgical interventions such as craniotomy [33, 150, 151], stereotactic [154], or radiosurgical procedures [48]. Noninvasive preoperative mapping is particularly important in view of the often aberrant anatomic layout of the brain mechanism for language functions associated with neurological disorders and brain damage [20, 150, 155–158].

Recording language-related magnetic fields (LRFs)

LRF sources

Long latency fields between 200 and 800 ms evoked by verbal stimuli that the patient is asked to process in a particular manner constitute the target MEG data. These fields are evoked regardless of stimulus modality – visual or auditory – and reflect neurophysiological activity produced during engagement of the brain mechanism responsible for processing them according to specific task requirements and instructions. In contrast to activity associated with the clinically relevant SEF sources, LRF testing requires that the patient maintain a high level of general alertness, focus on the stimuli, and perform the task adequately. Neurophysiological activity sampled by LRFs originates from several cortical regions in posterior temporal and – depending on the task – frontal cortices. LRF sources are computed throughout the late portion of the MEG-averaged waveform creating a (time) series of potentially useful brain-activation snapshots. The precise spatiotemporal profile of this activity varies greatly among individuals, patients and healthy participants alike, and special techniques have been developed to isolate clinically significant portions of this activity. The final product is a small set of active regions – often a single region – where LRF sources are observed with a high degree of intraindividual consistency. Depending on the activation task, these sources may be used to identify the location of receptive (Wernicke's area) or expressive language-specific (Broca's area) cortex. The degree of hemispheric asymmetry in the duration or strength of activation may also be used as an index of hemispheric dominance for language functions.

Stimulation

Language stimuli are presented using the same devices described in previous chapters of this section for AEFs and VEFs. Word stimuli are most frequently used in the context of both receptive and expressive language tasks. In one such procedure [159], patients are trained to recognize a set of 30 abstract, spoken English words. During the MEG recording session, six blocks of such stimuli are presented. Within each block of 40 words, 30 belong to the training set and 10 are novel distractors. The patient's task is to attend to, and indicate, via a manual response whether a word belongs to the training set. A sufficient number of blocks (usually 6) are presented allowing computation of two separate sets of LRFs (see the data processing section below). Kamada and colleagues [149] used a slightly different approach to ensure "deep" linguistic processing of word stimuli. They presented a list of 100 printed Kana words to their patients who were instructed to judge if each word had an abstract or concrete meaning. Bowyer and coworkers [148] used a verb-generation and a picture-naming task. A series of 100 concrete, high-frequency printed nouns were presented during the former task and patients were asked to silently derive appropriate verbs from each noun. The picture-naming task required patients to silently name a series of 100 black-and-white line drawings of everyday objects. To keep patients alert, investigators randomly interspersed distractor stimuli among targets in both tasks.

Patient alertness and cooperation

Language-related magnetic activity is affected by the level of alertness of the patient to an even higher degree than motor or early auditory evoked magnetic fields. Therefore, one must confirm that the participant has had adequate sleep on the night before the study. The occipital alpha rhythm in the ongoing MEG can be used to monitor wakefulness. During the study, the patient should be instructed to maintain eye fixation so that ocular artifacts and the occurrence of prominent alpha waves are reduced. Breaks should be allowed in order to reduce fatigue and eye blinking during the recording sessions.

Time should be allowed for the participant to practice the activation task. Depending on access to the neuromagnetometer system, practice can take place in the MEG shielded room or at a computer. Practicing the task is important for several reasons: (1) practice allows the participant to feel comfortable with the instructions so that, once begun, data collection would not need to be stopped and restarted due to confusion over the task; (2) amplitude effects occur when a person is exposed to stimuli for the first time, and during practice the participant can get comfortable with the testing environment, the stimuli, and the required responses prior to data collection. If the experiment incorporates a behavioral task, one might set a proportion of correct responses as a criterion to decide how long the subject practices the task during the practice session; for example, requiring that every participant reach a certain percent correct over a set number of trials prior to actually participating in the task during MEG recording. Additional criteria can be adopted requiring that each participant must reach a certain proportion of correct responses to be a good candidate for the MEG portion of the experiment.

Recording parameters

The typical recording session requires the patient to lie motionless on a bed with their head inside the helmet-like cavity of the dewar for approximately 15 minutes. The signal is filtered online with a band-pass between 0.1 and 20 to 30 Hz, digitized for 950 ms – at a minimum sampling rate of 254 Hz – including a 150 ms prestimulus period. On rare occasions when ambient magnetic noise is very prominent, the high-pass filter may be set to 1 Hz. Application of adaptive filtering algorithms is often necessary to further reduce the amount of low-frequency magnetic noise that is typically present in MEG recordings with relatively low high-pass filter settings.

Data processing

Artifact rejection should be rather rigorous and can be achieved through visual inspection of single-trial ERF segments to identify those contaminated by

(1) eye- or head-movement-related magnetic artifacts, or (2) epileptiform activity. Movement artifacts are defined as magnetic flux deflections in excess of 2 to 3 pT (picotesla) peak-to-peak in the recordings from magnetometer sensors located over the eyes. Since mistaking small blinks or conjugate eye movements with magnetic deflections caused by brain activation can occur, the surface distribution of magnetic flux associated with these deflections should be taken into account. LRF epochs that contain frequent, i.e., more than two, inter-ictal epileptiform events (spikes or sharp waves) may be excluded from further analyses. Examples of single-trial epochs recorded in the context of a language-mapping study are shown in Fig. 19.1 (Chapter 19) displaying various types of magnetic artifacts. Figure 24.1 shows examples of acceptable and unusable averaged LRFs.

Modeling intracranial sources as ECDs remains the most frequently used procedure to obtain cortical maps of task-related neurophysiological activation. The dipolar source(s) that account for the average surface distribution of magnetic flux at each 4-ms time window identify the brain areas activated at that time point. For a given point in time, the source-fitting algorithm is applied to the magnetic flux measurements obtained from a group of 34 to 38 sensors, always including both magnetic flux extrema. Auditory tasks are more suitable for this approach because associated contour maps tend to be dipolar for large portions of the averaged LRF epoch [159]. Source computation is restricted to latency periods during which one or two pairs of clearly distinct magnetic flux extrema are present over each side of the head. Source solutions are considered satisfactory if they are associated with a correlation coefficient of at least 0.9 between the observed and the "best" predicted magnetic field distribution and a confidence volume of 10 cm^3 or less. The derived activation maps consist of *clusters* of temporally contiguous activity sources that are typically localized in the same anatomical region. Clusters span between 20 and 100 ms in duration, although successive sources in the same region – usually temporoparietal cortex in the dominant hemisphere – lasting 400 ms or more are not uncommon. After dipole fitting, the estimated activity sources from the two recording sessions are merged and ranked by (1) the degree of latency overlap and (2) spatial proximity using an automated algorithm [159]. Complementary measures of the degree of regional activity are also examined, i.e., the peak global field power (RMS) and the peak current moment (Q). The method that produces the most conclusive results as an index of the degree of regional activation is the total *number* of successive activity sources in a particular area or group of areas. Note that none of the parameters of the early components are found to be predictive of Wada-based hemispheric dominance estimates.

More recently [160], a fully automated procedure for obtaining estimates of hemispheric dominance for language has been developed and validated using the data set originally reported by Papanicolaou and colleagues [159]. The procedure automates data preprocessing, noise reduction, artifact rejection,

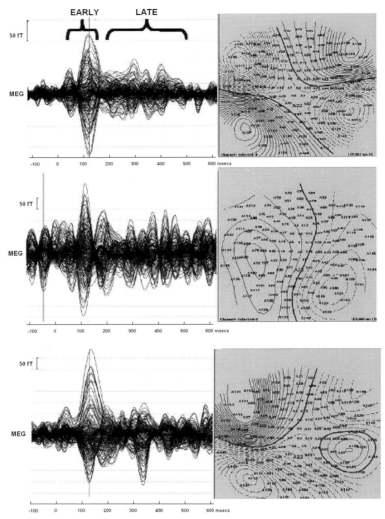

Fig. 24.1. Upper row: averaged LRF waveforms recorded from the entire set of 148 magnetometer sensors during a typical MEG recording session. The inset displays the isofield contour map of magnetic flux recorded at the peak of the auditory M100 response. Notice the symmetry between the left- and right-hemisphere maps. Middle row: an example of unacceptable MEG data due to excessive contamination by large amplitude rhythmic background activity (primarily in the alpha band, originating from occipital cortices, as the inset indicates). Lower row: a second example of unacceptable MEG data due to the presence of a significant lateral asymmetry in the amplitude of the M100 response ([left M100 RMS minus right M100 RMS]/[sum of left plus right M100 RMS] = >0.3). Unpublished data, MEG Laboratory, University of Texas Health Science Center at Houston.

and ECD fitting. The averaged data are first scanned for the presence of single dipolar distributions; the algorithm determines the channel grouping that best covers each such distribution and uses the portion of the flux distribution covered by such channel groupings to estimate the underlying dipolar source. Next, the single dipoles that account for surface dipolar maps are derived by the standard model [161], and the entire procedure is repeated at successive latency points until the entire EMF duration is exhausted. Finally, those dipolar sources that met the criteria of acceptability (correlation $\geq$ 0.9, confidence volume $\leq$ 20 cm^3) are retained, overlaid on the patient's MRI and used to determine hemispheric dominance in the same manner as manually derived ECDs.

Normative LRF data

An example of an averaged LRF record obtained with the procedures proposed by Papanicolaou and coworkers [142, 159] is shown in Fig. 24.2. The LRF typically consists of an early portion, typically between 30 and 200 ms poststimulus onset, and a late portion, typically between 200 and 800 ms poststimulus onset, although task-relevant activity up to 1000 ms may occasionally be observed. Contours at different time points show the presence of bilaterally symmetric dipolar distributions of magnetic flux during the early part of the epoch. Notice that with many patients, and especially children, the typical progression of maps from P50m to M100 to M200 may be absent.

Hemispheric dominance for language

The general approach to the estimation of hemispheric dominance for language, in most functional brain-imaging studies, has been to consider the degree of activation of each hemisphere during performance of a language task as an index of the degree of hemispheric engagement. The difference in activation levels between the hemispheres is then used to derive an estimate of hemispheric dominance.

In the context of the procedure introduced by Papanicolaou and associates [159, 160] the following are applied: (1) activity sources computed during the late portion of the LRF waveform for each hemisphere and testing session (i.e., $> \sim$200 ms) are selected; (2) the number of automatically clustered activity sources in perisylvian regions for each hemisphere and during each testing session, separately, is determined and counted; and (3) a laterality index is computed according to the formula: $(R-L)/(R+L)$, where R represents the number of acceptable late activity sources observed in the right hemisphere and L the corresponding number on the left. Index values between -0.1 and 0.1 were considered as indicative of bilaterally symmetric activation, whereas

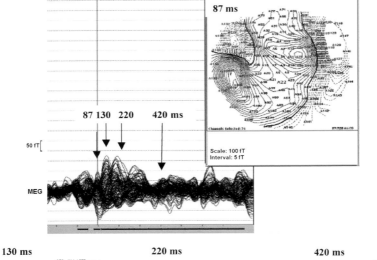

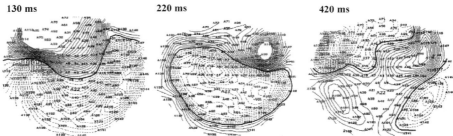

Fig. 24.2. Typical averaged LRF that was used for hemispheric dominance judgment using the protocol introduced by Papanicolaou and colleagues [159]. Arrows indicate latencies at which corresponding contour maps are shown below. Unpublished data, MEG Laboratory, University of Texas Health Science Center at Houston.

values > 0.1 or < −0.1 as indicative of right or left hemisphere dominance, respectively (see Fig. 24.3).

In the same study, concurrent validity estimates were calculated from a series of 100 consecutive patients, ranging in age from 8 to 56 years, who were evaluated for epilepsy surgery. When the above procedure was used, MEG and Wada tests exhibited complete agreement in 74 of 85 (87%) cases. Data from 11 cases were discordant. In the majority of the discordant cases ($n = 7$), MEG detected considerable activity in both hemispheres, although the Wada suggested left hemisphere dominance. In 4 of these 7 cases, the patients' epileptogenic zone was in the right hemisphere. A possible explanation for the discordance in these patients is that the degree of neurophysiological activation detected and successfully modeled from the right hemisphere was inflated by the presence of focal

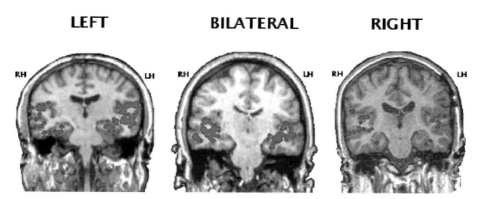

Fig. 24.3. Sample cortical activation maps obtained from three patients: A patient with left- (left column) and right-hemisphere dominance for language (right column), and a patient with bihemispheric representation of language function (middle column). Each of the coronal MRI slices displayed here contains a complete set of activity sources computed after the initial sensory activation (>200 ms poststimulus onset). Adapted from Papanicolaou and coworkers [159], with permission.

epileptiform activity that was not initially detected and therefore not rejected at the single-epoch level. The probability of discordant judgment did not appear to be related to location of seizure onset, seizure etiology, or handedness. MEG laterality judgments had an overall sensitivity of 0.98 and a lower selectivity of 0.83 because MEG detected more activity in the nondominant hemisphere than would be predicted by the results of the Wada procedure. Using identical stimulation and analysis procedures, Maestú and colleagues [147] replicated these results independently for Spanish-speaking patients. More recently, Merrifield and coworkers [162] reported similar results with a separate series of English-speaking epilepsy patients using slightly different acquisition and analysis procedures. Lee and associates [144], using the activation procedure developed by Papanicolaou and colleagues [159], reported interrater reliability in the estimation of hemispheric dominance for language as $r = 0.88$ in 21 surgical epilepsy candidates.

Kamada and colleagues [149], using similar recording and analysis procedures but a visual language task, reported an equivalent success rate for predicting hemispheric dominance for language in 117 patients suffering from tumors, AVMs, or medically intractable epilepsy. They reported successful mapping procedures in 85.4% of the patients. Failure to obtain useful LRF data was due mainly to excessive ocular artifacts in the group of epilepsy patients. Acceptable ECDs were found mostly in the posterior portion of the superior and middle temporal gyri and in adjacent inferior parietal cortices. Eighty-five patients were classified as left dominant, 11 as right dominant, and 3 as having bihemispheric distribution of the components of the brain mechanism for language. In the epilepsy group ($n = 31$), left hemispheric dominance was found in 84%; right, in 10%; and bihemispheric, in 6% of the patients. Corresponding percentages in the nonepilepsy group ($n = 68$) were 87%, 12%, and 1%, respectively. These results confirm the proportions of laterality judgements reported previously using similar tasks.

Functional mapping of the receptive and expressive language-specific cortex

The activation and data analysis protocol described in Papanicolaou and colleagues [159] yields reliable estimates of the location of receptive language-specific cortex (Wernicke's area), and the accuracy of these estimates has been verified against the results of invasive intra- or extraoperative electrocortical stimulation mapping [150, 151]. An example of the successful use of this procedure is presented in Fig. 24.4.

Test–retest reliability estimates for the location of Wernicke's area have been reported to average 0.8 cm (ranging from 0.2 to 0.8 cm) for healthy participants [163] and 0.75 cm (ranging from 0.3 to 0.9 cm) for epilepsy surgical candidates [144]. These values compare favorably to those obtained for somatosensory and early auditory EMF components.

Assessing hemispheric dominance for language can be accomplished by magnetic field mapping of the receptive language cortex, but can mapping LRFs determine the location of expressive language cortex in relation to diseased cortex? Several groups have thus far reported success in eliciting prefrontal magnetic activity in the vicinity of Broca's area, associated with the performance of a variety of expressive language tasks.

Castillo and coworkers [152] used a picture-naming task and MEG analysis procedures identical to those employed earlier in the context of receptive language mapping to derive maps of activation related to expressive language function. The results for 7 normal volunteers and 9 patients with epilepsy can be summarized as follows: (1) the task resulted in activation of the expressive language-specific cortex (Broca's area) in only a fraction of the cases (in 3 of the 9 patients and 3 of the 7 neurologically intact participants); (2) when prefrontal activity sources were identified, their location matched very closely with estimates of the location of Broca's area based on electrocortical stimulation mapping. (Based on his experience, this author notes that detection of activation in Broca's area is significantly improved with the use of a first-order gradiometer system with 248 sensors, instead of the 148-magnetometer system used by Castillo and coworkers.)

Kober and colleagues [75] also reported success in eliciting inferior frontal activity using a picture-naming task and spatial filtering rather than the single ECD method. The spatial localization and time-course results of the Kober

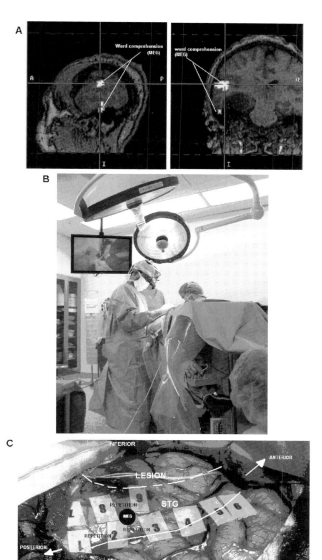

Fig. 24.4. (a) MEG/MSI-derived estimates of the location of receptive language-specific cortex in a patient with a large left temporal tumor. MEG identified two areas engaged during a word comprehension task (the left superior temporal gyrus and the left inferior temporal gyrus) in close proximity to the patient's lesion. (B) Intraoperative setting where electrocortical stimulation is conducted. (C) Digital picture of the exposed brain with landmarks indicating the borders of the lesion and areas where electrocortical stimulation produced errors in word comprehension and repetition (in close agreement with MEG/MSI-derived estimates). Unpublished data, MEG Laboratory, University of Texas Health Science Center at Houston.

group were consistent with the Wernicke–Geschwind model of language organization. Moreover, they showed a high degree of concordance between results from spatial filtering and single ECD modeling.

Bowyer and coworkers [164], using yet another mathematical procedure for estimating the underlying cortical sources of magnetic fields – namely, multiresolution (MR)-FOCUSS – showed in a group of 24 epileptic patients and 18 control subjects that this current-density imaging technique can provide reasonable localization of language cortex. When this technique is used, all participants showed activation of the left superior temporal gyrus during a word-generation task and of the left inferior frontal gyrus during a picture-naming task. Although the spatial filtering and current source density methods have not been externally validated for language mapping against the Wada procedure or electrocortical stimulation mapping, they hold promise for detecting multiple, simultaneous sources contributing to late components of event-related fields during expressive and receptive language tasks. Moreover, Bowyer and colleagues [153] collected MEG data during the verb-generation and picture-naming tasks from 27 patients with medically intractable epilepsy, all of whom also received the Wada test. The investigators determined the location and extent of neurophysiological activation using the MR-FOCUSS algorithm, from which they calculated a laterality index. The laterality indices (LIs) for three separate latencies, within each language task, were calculated to determine the latency that correlated best with each patient's Wada result. The LI for all language processing was calculated for the interval 150 to 550 ms, the second LI was calculated for the interval 230 to 290 ms (Wernicke's area of activation), and the third LI was calculated for the interval 396 to 460 ms (Broca's area of activation). In 23 of 24 epilepsy patients with a successful Wada test, the LIs for activation of Broca's area during the picture-naming task were in agreement with the results of the Wada (96% agreement). One of 3 patients who had an undetermined or bilateral Wada test outcome had an LI calculated for activation of Broca's area (396 to 460 ms) that agreed with intracranial mapping and clinical testing. These results suggest an 89% agreement rate (24 of 27) for MEG/MSI LI determination of the language-dominant hemisphere. Promising results in the same direction have also been reported by Hirata and coworkers [165], using a different algorithm for source estimation. Oscillatory activity associated with reading was recorded in 20 patients and was in agreement with the results of the Wada test.

Aberrant LRFs

MEG-derived estimates of late neurophysiological activation during the processing of language stimuli is used to explore the potentially aberrant organization of the brain mechanisms that support language functions in developmental disorders (autism, early-onset epileptic syndromes) and following acquired brain lesions (stroke, late-onset focal epilepsy).

Functional reorganization of the brain as a result of acquired focal lesions involving language-specific cortex have been observed in several cases and documented with MEG/MSI. In one of the few large patient series reported [157], patients with medically intractable epilepsy arising from the left temporal lobe showed significantly higher frequency of atypical lateralization of language – either right-hemisphere dominance or bilateral language representation – compared with patients sustaining left-hemisphere focal lesions (43% vs. 13%, respectively). In fact, the majority of patients who experienced early seizure onset (before 5 years of age) showed atypical lateralization of language. In contrast, the precise location of cortex involved in language comprehension, within the dominant hemisphere, was found to be atypical (outside of Wernicke's area) in 30% of patients with focal lesions, but in only 14% of the epilepsy patients, who also showed significant degeneration of the mesial temporal lobe. These findings indicate an increased probability that a partial or total shift of the brain mechanism responsible for language comprehension to the nondominant hemisphere in patients with mesial temporal lobe epilepsy occurred.

In a subsequent study, reorganization of the brain mechanisms for language comprehension as a result of resection of the anterior portion of the left temporal lobe was investigated [166]. Patients with atypical (bilateral) language lateralization, according to both the Wada procedure and preoperative MEG/MSI, were significantly more likely than patients with left-hemisphere dominance to show a shift in language representation toward greater right-hemispheric involvement after surgery. Conversely, patients with left-hemispheric dominance preoperatively were more likely to show intrahemispheric changes involving a slight inferior shift of the putative location of Wernicke's area. Patients with bilateral representation tended to perform worse on neuropsychological test measures pre- and postoperatively (see also [158]). These preliminary findings show that MEG/MSI can contribute significantly not only to the localization of Wernicke's area for presurgical planning, but may also serve as an important tool for documenting postoperative intra- and interhemispheric language reorganization trends.

Potential indices of reorganization of the brain mechanisms for language functions in patients who developed aphasia following left-hemisphere CVAs have also been studied. For instance, Breier and coworkers [167] tested 6 patients who had suffered left middle-cerebral-artery stroke on the word-recognition task described above [159]. As expected, patients exhibited relatively decreased activation in areas known to be involved in the receptive language function, including the left superior temporal gyrus, as well as increased activation of areas outside this region that might potentially support language function. In a subsequent study, patients who responded well to constraint-induced language therapy exhibited a greater degree of late MEG activation in posterior language areas of the left hemisphere and homotopic areas of the right hemisphere prior to therapy than those who did not respond well [168]. Response to therapy, however, was positively correlated with the degree of pretherapy MEG activity within posterior areas of the right hemisphere only on an individual basis.

25

Alternative techniques for evoked magnetic field data – future directions

Spectral analysis of MEG data

In parallel to the analysis of ERFs, the frequency domain of MEG data can be explored in terms of power at single-sensor locations or functional coupling between pairs of sensors (or pairs of sources).

Event-related desynchronization (ERD) and event-related synchronization (ERS)

ERD and ERS of EEG or MEG rhythms describe neuroelectric events preceding and following a task execution [169–171]. ERD/ERS may reveal a reduction or increase in EEG power during an event – sensory, cognitive, motor – when compared to baseline at a certain frequency band.

Temporal spectral evolution (TSE)

An alternative procedure frequently used for MEG data is the TSE analysis, which provides an index of event-related changes in the magnitude of the magnetic fields in the physical unit of the recording [172].

Coherence

The functional coupling of brain rhythms, spectral coherence analysis indexes the temporal synchronization of two EEG or MEG time series (i.e., relative to two sensors), in frequency domain (i.e., frequency-by-frequency), and helps to assess linear functional cortico-cortical connectivity. In general, decreased coherence indices reduce linear functional connections and information transfer (i.e., uncoupling) between cortical areas beneath the paired electrodes or modulation of common areas by a third region. In contrast, increased coherence augments linear functional connections and information transfer (i.e., coupling), which reflects a functional interaction of different cortical-draftrules structures for a given task.

Direct transfer function (DTF)

Finally, the direction of the information flow within the coupled EEG rhythms can be estimated by the DTF approach [173, 174].

References

1. Orrison WW, Davis LE, Sullivan GW, Mettler FA Jr, Flynn ER. Anatomic localization of cerebral cortical function by magnetoencephalography combined with MR imaging and CT. *Am J Neuroradiol* 1990; **11**(4): 713–716.
2. Orrison WW Jr, Rose DF, Hart BL, *et al*. Noninvasive preoperative cortical localization by magnetic source imaging. *Am J Neuroradiol* 1992; **13**(4): 1124–1128.
3. Gallen CC, Sobel DF, Waltz T, *et al*. Noninvasive presurgical neuromagnetic mapping of somatosensory cortex. *Neurosurgery* 1993; **33**(2): 260–268.
4. Smith JR, Gallen C, Orrison W, *et al*. Role of multichannel magnetoencephalography in the evaluation of ablative seizure surgery candidates. *Stereotact Funct Neurosurg* 1994; **62**(1–4): 238–244.
5. Nakasato N, Fujita S, Seki K, *et al*. Functional localization of bilateral auditory cortices using an MRI-linked whole head magnetoencephalography (MEG) system. *Electroenceph Clin Neurophysiol* 1995; **94**(3): 183–190.
6. Rezai AR, Mogilner AY, Cappell J, Hund M, Llinas RR, Kelly PJ. Integration of functional brain mapping in image-guided neurosurgery. *Acta Neurochir Suppl* (Wien) 1997; **68**: 85–89.
7. Kamada K, Oshiro O, Takeuchi F, *et al*. Identification of central sulcus by using somatosensory evoked magnetic fields and brain surface MR images: three dimensional projection analysis. *J Neurol Sci* 1993; **116**(1): 29–33.
8. Nakamura A, Yamada T, Goto A, *et al*. Somatosensory homunculus as drawn by MEG. *NeuroImage* 1998; **7**(4): 377–386.
9. Ishibashi H, Morioka T, Nishio S, Shigeto H, Yamamoto T, Fukui M. Magnetoencephalographic investigation of somatosensory homunculus in patients with peri-Rolandic tumors. *Neurol Res* 2001; **23**(1): 29–38.
10. Nagamatsu K, Nakasato N, Hatanaka K, Kanno A, Iwasaki M, Yoshimoto T. Neuromagnetic detection and localization of N15, the initial response to trigeminal stimulus. *Neuroreport* 2001; **12**(1): 1–5.
11. Morioka T, Yamamoto T, Katsuta T, Fujii K, Fukui M. Presurgical three-dimensional magnetic source imaging of the somatosensory cortex in a patient with a peri-Rolandic lesion: technical note. *Neurosurgery* 1994; **34**(5): 930–933.
12. Gallen CC, Schwartz BJ, Bucholz RD, *et al*. Presurgical localization of functional cortex using magnetic source imaging. *J Neurosurg* 1995; **82**(6): 988–994.
13. Roberts TP, Zusman E, McDermott M, Barbaro N, Rowley HA. Correlation of functional magnetic source imaging with intraoperative cortical stimulation in neurosurgical patients. *J Image Guid Surg* 1995; **1**(6): 339–347.

14. Morioka T, Shigeto H, Ishibashi H, *et al.* Magnetic source imaging of the sensory cortex on the surface anatomy MR scanning. *Neurol Res* 1998; **20**(3): 235–241.

15. Nimsky C, Ganslandt O, Kober H, *et al.* Integration of functional magnetic resonance imaging supported by magnetoencephalography in functional neuronavigation. *Neurosurgery* 1999; **44**(6): 1249–1255.

16. Roberts TP, Ferrari P, Perry D, Rowley HA, Berger MS. Presurgical mapping with magnetic source imaging: comparisons with intraoperative findings. *Brain Tumor Pathol* 2000; **17**(2): 57–64.

17. Schiffbauer H, Berger MS, Ferrari P, Freudenstein D, Rowley HA, Roberts TP. Preoperative magnetic source imaging for brain tumor surgery: a quantitative comparison with intraoperative sensory and motor mapping. *J Neurosurg* 2002; **97**(6): 1333–1342.

18. Iwasaki M, Nakasato N, Kanno A, *et al.* Somatosensory evoked fields in patients with comatose survivors after severe head injury. *Clin Neurophysiol* 2001; **112**(1): 204–210.

19. Ishitobi M, Nakasato N, Yoshimoto T, Iinuma K. Abnormal primary somatosensory function in unilateral polymicrogyria: an MEG study. *Brain Dev* 2005; **27**(1): 22–29.

20. Papanicolaou AC, Simos PG, Breier JI, *et al.* Brain plasticity for sensory and linguistic functions: a functional imaging study using magnetoencephalography with children and young adults. *J Child Neurol* 2001; **16**(4): 241–252.

21. Vates GE, Lawton MT, Wilson CB, *et al.* Magnetic source imaging demonstrates altered cortical distribution of function in patients with arteriovenous malformations. *Neurosurgery* 2002; **51**(3): 614–627.

22. Oishi M, Fukuda M, Kameyama S, Kawaguchi T, Masuda H, Tanaka R. Magnetoencephalographic representation of the sensorimotor hand area in cases of intracerebral tumour. *J Neurosurg Psychiatry* 2003; **74**(12): 1649–1654.

23. Lewine JD, Astur RS, Davis LE, Knight JE, Maclin EL, Orrison WW Jr. Cortical organization in adulthood is modified by neonatal infarct: a case study. *Radiology* 1994; **190**(1): 93–96.

24. Breier JI, Simos PG, Zouridakis G, *et al.* A MEG study of cortical plasticity. *Neurocase* 1999; **5**: 277–284.

25. Burneo JG, Kuzniecky RI, Bebin M, Knowlton RC. Cortical reorganization in malformations of cortical development: a magnetoencephalographic study. *Neurology* 2004; **63**(10): 1818–1824.

26. Rossini PM, Caltagirone C, Castriota-Scanderbeg A, *et al.* Hand motor cortical area reorganization in stroke: a study with fMRI, MEG and TCS maps. *Neuroreport* 1998; **9**(9): 2141–2146.

27. Rossini PM, Tecchio F, Pizzella V, *et al.* On the reorganization of sensory hand areas after mono-hemispheric lesion: a functional (MEG)/anatomical (MRI) integrative study. *Brain Res* 1998; **782**(1–2): 153–166.

28. Rossini PM, Tecchio F, Pizzella V, Lupoi D, Cassetta E, Paqualetti P. Interhemispheric differences of sensory hand areas after monohemispheric stroke: MEG/MRI integrative study. *NeuroImage* 2001; **14**(2): 474–485.

29. Druschky K, Kaltenhauser M, Hummel C, *et al.* Post-apoplectic reorganization of cortical areas processing passive movement and tactile stimulation – a neuromagnetic case study. *Neuroreport* 2002; **13**(18): 2581–2586.

30. Ossenblok P, Leijten FS, de Munck JC, Huiskamp GJ, Barkhof F, Boon P. Magnetic source imaging contributes to the presurgical identification of sensorimotor cortex in patients with frontal lobe epilepsy. *Clin Neurophysiol* 2003; **114**(2): 221–232.

31. Ganslandt O, Steinmeier R, Kober H, *et al.* Magnetic source imaging combined with image-guided frameless stereotaxy: a new method in surgery around the motor strip. *Neurosurgery* 1997; **41**(3): 621–627.

32. Castillo EM, Simos PG, Wheless JW, *et al.* Integrating sensory and motor mapping in a comprehensive MEG protocol: clinical validity and replicability. *NeuroImage* 2004; **21**(3): 973–983.

33. Ganslandt O, Buchfelder M, Hastreiter P, Grummich P, Fahlbusch R, Nimsky C. Magnetic source imaging supports clinical decision making in glioma patients. *Clin Neurol Neurosurg* 2004; **107**(1): 20–26.

34. Shimamura N, Ohkuma H, Ogane K, *et al.* Displacement of central sulcus in cerebral arteriovenous malformation situated in the peri-motor cortex as assessed by magnetoencephalographic study. *Acta Neurochir* (Wien) 2004; **146**(4): 363–368.

35. Rezai AR, Hund M, Kronberg E, *et al.* The interactive use of magnetoencephalography in stereotactic image-guided neurosurgery. *Neurosurgery* 1996; **39**(1): 92–102.

36. Hund M, Rezai AR, Kronberg E, *et al.* Magnetoencephalographic mapping: basic of a new functional risk profile in the selection of patients with cortical brain lesions. *Neurosurgery* 1997; **40**(5): 936–942.

37. Ganslandt O, Fahlbusch R, Nimsky C, *et al.* Functional neuronavigation with magnetoencephalography: outcome in 50 patients with lesions around the motor cortex. *J Neurosurg* 1999; **91**(1): 73–79.

38. McDonald JD, Chong BW, Lewine JD, *et al.* Integration of preoperative and intraoperative functional brain mapping in a frameless stereotactic environment for lesions near eloquent cortex. Technical note. *J Neurosurg* 1999; **90**(3): 591–598.

39. Alberstone CD, Skirboll SL, Benzel EC, *et al.* Magnetic source imaging and brain surgery: presurgical and intraoperative planning in 26 patients. *J Neurosurg* 2000; **92**(1): 79–90.

40. Fahlbusch R, Ganslandt O, Nimsky C. Intraoperative imaging with open magnetic resonance imaging and neuronavigation. *Childs Nerv Syst* 2000; **16**(10–11): 829–831.

41. Mäkelä JP, Kirveskari E, Seppa M, *et al.* Three-dimensional integration of brain anatomy and function to facilitate intraoperative navigation around the sensorimotor strip. *Hum Brain Mapp* 2001; **12**(3): 180–192.

42. Firsching R, Bondar I, Heinze HJ, *et al.* Practicability of magnetoencephalography-guided neuronavigation. *Neurosurg Rev* 2002; **25**(1–2): 73–78.

43. Jannin P, Morandi X, Fleig OJ, *et al.* Integration of sulcal and functional information for multimodal neuronavigation. *J Neurosurg* 2002; **96**(4): 713–723.

44. Kamada K, Houkin K, Takeuchi F, *et al.* Visualization of the eloquent motor system by integration of MEG, functional, and anisotropic diffusion-weighted MRI in functional neuronavigation. *Surg Neurol* 2003; **59**(5): 352–361.

45. Kamiryo T, Cappell J, Kronberg E, *et al.* Interactive use of cerebral angiography and magnetoencephalography in arteriovenous malformations: technical note. *Neurosurgery* 2002; **50**(4): 903–911.

46. Yang TT, Gallen CC, Ramachandran VS, Cobb S, Schwartz BJ, Bloom FE. Non-invasive detection of cerebral plasticity in adult human somatosensory cortex. *Neuroreport* 1994; **5**(6): 701–704.

47. Aoyama H, Kamada K, Shirato H, *et al.* Visualization of the corticospinal tract pathway using magnetic resonance axonography and magnetoencephalography for stereotactic irradiation planning of arteriovenous malformations. *Radiother Oncol* 2003; **68**(1): 27–32.

48. Aoyama H, Kamada K, Shirato H, *et al.* Integration of functional brain information into stereotactic irradiation treatment planning using magnetoencephalography and magnetic resonance axonography. *Int J of Radiat Oncol Biol Phys* 2004; **58**(4): 1177–1183.

49. Elbert T, Candia V, Altenmuller E, *et al.* Alteration of digital representations in somatosensory cortex in focal hand dystonia. *Neuroreport* 1998; **9**(16): 3571–3575.

50. Theuvenet PJ, Dunajski Z, Peters MJ, van Ree JM. Responses to median and tibial nerve stimulation in patients with chronic neuropathic pain. *Brain Topogr* 1999; **11**(4): 305–313.

51. Druschky K, Kaltenhauser M, Hummel C, *et al.* Alteration of the somatosensory cortical map in peripheral mononeuropathy due to carpal tunnel syndrome. *Neuroreport* 2000; **11**(17): 3925–3930.

52. Meunier S, Garnero L, Ducorps A, *et al.* Human brain mapping in dystonia reveals both endophenotypic traits and adaptive reorganization. *Ann Neurol* 2001; **50**(4): 521–527.

53. Tecchio F, Padua L, Aprile I, Rossini PM. Carpal tunnel syndrome modifies sensory hand cortical somatotopy: A MEG study. *Hum Brain Mapp* 2002; **17**(1): 28–36.

54. Mertens M, Lütkenhöner B. Efficient neuromagnetic determination of landmarks in the somatosensory cortex. *Clin Neurophysiol* 2000; **111**: 1478–1487.

55. Simoes C, Mertens M, Forss N, Jousmaki V, Lütkenhöner B, Hari R. Functional overlap of finger representations in human SI and SII cortices. *J Neurophysiol* 2001; **86**: 1661–1665.

56. Nevalainen P, Ramstad R, Isotalo E, Haapanen M-L, Lauronen L. Trigeminal somatosensory evoked magnetic fields to tactile stimulation. *Clin Neurophysiol* 2006; **117**: 2007–2015.

57. Itomi K, Kakigi R, Maeda K, Hoshiyama M. Dermatome versus homunculus: detailed topography of the primary somatosensory cortex following trunk stimulation. *Clin Neurophysiol* 2000; **111**(3): 405–412.

58. Castillo EM, Papanicolaou AC. Cortical representation of dermatomes: MEG-derived maps after tactile stimulation. *NeuroImage* 2005; **25**(3): 727–733.

59. Lin YY, Chen WT, Liao KK, *et al.* Differential generators for N20m and P35m responses to median nerve stimulation. *NeuroImage* 2005; **25**(4): 1090–1099.

60. Bercovici E, Pang EW, Sharma R, *et al.* Somatosensory-evoked fields on magnetoencephalography for epilepsy infants younger than 4 years with total intravenous anesthesia. *Clin Neurophysiol* 2008; **119**(6): 1328–1334.

61. Kitamura Y, Kakigi R, Hoshiyama M, Koyama S, Nakamura A. Effects of sleep on somatosensory evoked responses in human: a magnetoencephalographic study. *Brain Res* 1996; **4**(4): 275–279.

62. Pikho E, Sambeth A, Leppänen PH, Okada Y, Lauronen L. Auditory evoked magnetic fields to speech stimuli in newborns – effect of sleep stages. *Neurol Clin Neurophysiol* 2004; **2004**: 6.

63. Stephen JM, Ranken D, Best E, *et al.* Aging changes and gender differences in response to median nerve stimulation measured with MEG. *Clin Neurophysiol* 2006; **117**(1): 131–143.

64. Lauronen L, Nevalainen P, Wikstrom H, Parkkonen L, Okada Y, Pihko E. Immaturity of somatosensory cortical processing in human newborns. *NeuroImage* 2006; **33**(1): 195–203.

65. Inoue K, Shirai T, Nakanishi K, *et al.* Difference in somatosensory evoked fields elicited by mechanical and electrical stimulations: elucidation of the human homunculus by a noninvasive method. *Hum Brain Mapp* 2005; **24**: 274–283.

66. Hoshiyama M, Kakigi R, Koyama S, Kitamura Y, Shimojo M, Watanabe S. Somatosensory evoked magnetic fields following stimulation of the lip in humans. *Electroencephalogr Clin Neurophysiol* 1996; **100**: 96–104.

67. Schaefer M, Rothemund Y, Heinze HJ, Rotte M. Short-term plasticity of the primary somatosensory cortex during tool use. *Neuroreport* 2004; **15**(8): 1293–1297.

68. Bast T, Wright T, Boor R, *et al.* Combined EEG and MEG analysis of early somatosensory evoked activity in children and adolescents with focal epilepsies. *Clin Neurophysiol* 2007; **118**(8): 1721–1735.

69. Roberts TP, Tran Q, Ferrari P, Berger MS. Increased somatosensory neuromagnetic fields ipsilateral to lesions in neurosurgical patients. *Neuroreport* 2002; **13**(5): 699–702.

70. Mima T, Nagamine T, Nakamura K, Shibasaki H. Attention modulates both primary and second somatosensory cortical activities in humans: a magnetoencephalographic study. *J Neurophysiol* 1998; **80**(4): 2215–2221.

71. Bundo M, Inao S, Nakamura A, *et al.* Changes of neural activity correlate with the severity of cortical ischemia in patients with unilateral major cerebral artery occlusion. *Stroke* 2002; **3**: 61–66.

72. Gaillen P, Aghulon C, Durufle A, *et al.* Magnetoencephalography in stroke: a 1-year follow-up study. *Eur J Neurol* 2003; **10**(4): 373–382.

73. Tecchio F, Zappasodi F, Tombini M, *et al.* Brain plasticity in recovery from stroke: an MEG assessment. *NeuroImage* 2006; **32**(3): 1326–1334.

74. Willemse RB, de Munck JC, van't Ent D, *et al.* Magnetoencephalographic study of posterior tibial nerve stimulation in patients with intracranial lesions around the central sulcus. *Neurosurgery* 2007; **61**(6): 1209–1217.

75. Kober H, Moller M, Nimsky C, Vieth J, Fahlbusch R, Ganslandt O. New approach to localize speech relevant brain areas and hemispheric dominance using spatially filtered magnetoencephalography. *Hum Brain Mapp* 2001; **14**(4): 236–250.

76. Minassian BA, Otsubo H, Weiss S, Elliott I, Rutka JT, Snead OC III. Magnetoencephalographic localization in pediatric epilepsy surgery: comparison with invasive intracranial electroencephalography. *Ann Neurol* 1999; **46**(4): 627–633.

77. Romstock J, Fahlbusch R, Ganslandt O, Nimsky C, Strauss C. Localisation of the sensorimotor cortex during surgery for brain tumours: feasibility and waveform

patterns of somatosensory evoked potentials. *J Neurol Neurosurg Psychiatry* 2002; **72**: 221–229.

78. Schiffbauer H, Ferrari P, Rowley HA, Berger MS, Roberts TP. Functional activity within brain tumors: a magnetic source imaging study. *Neurosurgery* 2001; **49**(6): 1313–1320.
79. Schulder M, Maldjian JA, Liu WC, *et al.* Functional image-guided surgery of intracranial tumors located in or near the sensorimotor cortex. *J Neurosurg* 1998; **89**(3): 412–418.
80. Deecke L, Boschert J, Weinberg H, Brickett P. Magnetic fields of the human brain (Bereitschaftmagnetfeld) preceding voluntary foot and toe movements. *Exp Brain Res* 1983; **52**: 81–96.
81. Nagamine T, Toro C, Balish M, *et al.* Cortical magnetic and electric fields associated with voluntary finger movements. *Brain Topogr* 1994; **6**(3): 175–183.
82. Hashimoto I, Mashiko T, Odaka K, Imada T, Mizuta T, Tomarikawa K. Bilateral activation of the human motor cortex preceding unilateral voluntary finger extension as evidenced by magnetic measurements. In: Baumgartner C, Deecke L, Stroink G, Williamson SJ, eds. *Biomagnetism: Fundamental Research and Clinical Applications.* Amsterdam: Elsevier. 1995; 131–135.
83. Hoshiyama M, Kakigi R, Berg P, *et al.* Identification of motor and sensory brain activities during unilateral finger movement: spatio-temporal source analysis of movement associated magnetic fields. *Exp Brain Res* 1997; **115**(1): 6–14.
84. Gerloff C, Uenishi N, Nagamine T, Kunieda T, Hallett M, Shibasaki H. Cortical activation during fast repetitive finger movements in humans: steady-state movement-related magnetic fields and their cortical generators. *Electroenceph Clin Neurophysiol* 1998; **109**(5): 444–453.
85. Taniguchi M, Yoshimine T, Cheyne D, *et al.* Neuromagnetic fields preceding unilateral movements in dextrals and sinistrals. *Neuroreport* 1998; **9**(7): 1497–1502.
86. Praamstra P, Schmitz F, Freund HJ, Schnitzler A. Magneto-encephalographic correlates of the lateralized readiness potential. *Brain Res* 1999; **8**(2): 77–85.
87. Nakasato N, Itoh H, Hatanaka K, Nakahara H, Kanno A, Yoshimoto T. Movement-related magnetic fields to tongue protrusion. *NeuroImage* 2001; **14**(4): 924–935.
88. Morioka T, Mizushima A, Yamamoto T, *et al.* Functional mapping of the sensorimotor cortex: combined use of magnetoencephalography, functional MRI, and motor evoked potentials. *Neuroradiology* 1995; **37**(7): 526–530.
89. Cheyne D, Endo H, Takeda T, Weinberg H. Sensory feedback contributes to early movement-evoked fields during voluntary finger movements in humans. *Brain Res* 1997; **771**(2): 196–202.
90. Lin PT, Berger MS, Nagarajan SS. Motor field sensitivity for preoperative localization of motor cortex. *J Neurosurg* 2006; **105**(4): 588–594.
91. Rosburg T, Weiss T, Haueisen J, Nowak H, Sauer H. Internal consistency of dipole localizations for the human movement-evoked magnetic field component 1 (MEF 1). *Neurosci Lett* 1996; **215**: 45–48.
92. Kirsch HE, Zhu Z, Honma S, Findlay A, Berger MS, Nagarajan SS. Predicting the location of mouth motor cortex in patients with brain tumors by using somatosensory evoked field measurements. *J Neurosurg* 2007; **107**(3): 481–487.

93. Kanno A, Nakasato N, Fujita S, *et al*. Right hemispheric dominance in the auditory evoked magnetic fields for pure-tone stimuli. *Electroenceph Clin Neurophysiol*, 1996; **47**(Suppl): 129–132.
94. Suzuki K, Okuda J, Nakasato N, *et al*. Auditory evoked magnetic fields in patients with right hemisphere language dominance. *Neuroreport* 1997; **8**(15): 3363–3366.
95. Kanno A, Nakasato N, Murayama N, Yoshimoto T. Middle and long latency peak sources in auditory magnetic fields for tone burst in humans. *Neurosci Lett* 2000; **293**(3): 187–190.
96. Nakasato N, Kumabe T, Kanno A, Ohtomo S, Mizoi K, Yoshimoto T. Neuromagnetic evaluation of cortical auditory function in patients with temporal lobe tumors. *J Neurosurg* 1997; **86**(4): 610–618.
97. Ohtomo S, Nakasato N, Kanno A, *et al*. Hemispheric asymmetry of the auditory evoked N100m response in relation to the crossing point between the central sulcus and sylvian fissure. *Electroenceph Clin Neurophysiol* 1998; **108**(3): 219–225.
98. Mäkelä JP, Hari R, Valanne L, Ahonen A. Auditory evoked magnetic fields after ischemic brain lesions. *Ann Neurol* 1991; **30**(1): 76–82.
99. Nakasato N, Yoshimoto T. Somatosensory, auditory, and visual evoked magnetic fields in patients with brain diseases. *J Clin Neurophysiol* 2000; **17**(2): 201–211.
100. Fujiki N, Naito Y, Nagamine T, *et al*. Influence of unilateral deafness on auditory evoked magnetic field. *Neuroreport* 1998; **9**(14): 3129–3133.
101. Toyoda K, Ibayashi S, Yamamoto T, Kuwabara Y, Fujishima M. Auditory evoked neuromagnetic response in cerebrovascular diseases: a preliminary study. *J Neurol Neurosurg Psychiatry* 1998; **64**(6): 777–784.
102. Dietrich V, Nieschalk M, Stoll W, Rajan R, Pantev C. Cortical reorganization in patients with high frequency cochlear hearing loss. *Hear Res* 2001; **158**(1–2): 95–101.
103. Kandori A, Oe H, Miyashita K, *et al*. Abnormal auditory neural networks in patients with right hemispheric infarction, chronic dizziness, and moyamoya disease: a magnetoencephalogram study. *Neurosci Res* 2002; **44**(3): 273–283.
104. Morita T, Naito Y, Nagamine T, Fujiki N, Shibasaki H, Ito J. Enhanced activation of the auditory cortex in patients with inner-ear hearing impairment: a magnetoencephalographic study. *Clin Neurophysiol* 2003; **114**(5): 851–859.
105. Teale P, Carlson J, Rojas D, Reite M. Reduced laterality of the source locations for generators of the auditory steady-state field in schizophrenia. *Biol Psychiatry* 2003; **54**(11): 1149–1153.
106. Paetau R, Saraneva J, Salonen O, Valanne L, Ignatius J, Salenius S. Electromagnetic function of polymicrogyric cortex in congenital bilateral perisylvian syndrome. *J Neurol Neurosurg Psychiatry* 2004; **75**(5): 717–722.
107. Pantev C, Hoke M, Lehnertz K, Lutkenhoner B, Fahrendorf G, Stober U. Identification of sources of brain neuronal activity with high spatiotemporal resolution through combination of neuromagnetic source localization (NMSL) and magnetic resonance imaging (MRI). *Electroencephalogr Clin Neurophysiol* 1990; **75**(3): 173–184.
108. Papanicolaou AC, Baumann S, Rogers RL, Saydjari C, Amparo EG, Eisenberg HM. Localization of auditory response sources using magnetoencephalography and magnetic resonance imaging. *Arch Neurol* 1990; **47**(1): 33–37.

109. Godey B, Schwartz D, de Graaf JB, Chauvel P, Liégeois-Chauvel C. Neuromagnetic source localization of auditory evoked fields and intracerebral evoked potentials: a comparison of data in the same patients. *Clin Neurophysiol* 2001; **112**: 1850–1859.

110. Takeshita K, Nagamine T, Thuy DH, *et al.* Maturational change of parallel auditory processing in school-aged children revealed by simultaneous recording of magnetic and electric cortical responses. *Clin Neurophysiol* 2002; **113**(9): 1470–1484.

111. Pantev C, Lutkenhoner B, Hoke M, Lehnertz K. Comparison between simultaneously recorded auditory-evoked magnetic fields and potentials elicited by ipsilateral, contralateral and binaural tone burst stimulation. *Audiology* 1986; **25**(1): 54–61.

112. Huotilainen M, Kujala A, Hotakainen M, Shestakova A, Kushnerenko E, Parkkonen L. Auditory magnetic responses of healthy newborns. *Neuroreport* 2003; **14**: 1871–1875.

113. Lutter WJ, Maier M, Wakai RT. Development of MEG sleep patterns and magnetic auditory evoked responses during early infancy. *Clin Neurophysiol* 2006; **117**: 522–530.

114. Pang EW, Gaetz W, Otsubo H, Chuang S, Cheyne D. Localization of auditory N1 in children using MEG: source modeling issues. *Int J Psychophysiol* 2003; **51**: 27–35.

115. Zouridakis G, Simos PG, Papanicolaou AC. Multiple bilaterally asymmetric cortical sources account for the auditory N1m component. *Brain Topogr* 1998; **10**(3): 183–189.

116. Virtanen J, Ahveninen J, Ilmoniemi RJ, Naatanen R, Pekkonen E. Replicability of MEG and EEG measures of the auditory N1/N1m-response. *Electroencephalogr Clin Neurophysiol* 1998; **108**(3): 291–298.

117. Mäkelä JP. Auditory evoked magnetic fields in stroke. *Physiol Meas* 1993; **14**(Suppl 4A): A51–A54.

118. Kubota Y, Otsuki T, Kaneko Y, Niimura K, Nakama H, Okazaki M. Delayed N100m latency in focal epilepsy associated with spike dipoles at the primary auditory cortex. *J Clin Neurophysiol* 2007; **24**(3): 263–270.

119. Mizuno T, Takanashi Y, Nakase T, *et al.* Clinical application of magnetoencephalography in a patient with corticobasal degeneration. *J Neuroimaging* 1999; **9**(1): 45–47.

120. Parviainen T, Helenius P, Salmelin R. Cortical differentiation of speech and non-speech sounds at 100 ms: implications for dyslexia. *Cereb Cortex* 2005; **15**(7): 1054–1063.

121. Heim S, Eulitz C, Elbert T. Altered hemispheric asymmetry of auditory P100m in dyslexia. *Eur J Neurosci* 2003; **17**(8): 1715–1722.

122. Gage NM, Siegel B, Callen M, Roberts TP. Cortical sound processing in children with autism disorder: an MEG investigation. *Neuroreport* 2003; **14**(16): 2047–2051.

123. Oram Cardy JE, Flagg EJ, Roberts W, Brian J, Roberts TP. Magnetoencephalography identifies rapid temporal processing deficit in autism and language impairment. *Neuroreport* 2005; **16**(4): 329–332.

124. Seki K, Nakasato N, Fujita S, *et al.* Neuromagnetic evidence that the P100 component of pattern reversal visual evoked response originates in the bottom of calcarine fissure. *Electroenceph Clin Neurophysiol* 1996; **100**(5): 436–442.

125. Nakamura A, Kakigi R, Hoshiyama M, Koyama S, Kitamura Y, Shimojo M. Visual evoked cortical magnetic fields to pattern reversal stimulation. *Cogn Brain Res* 1997; **6**: 9–22.

126. Portin K, Vanni S, Virsu V, Hari R. Stronger occipital cortical activation to lower than upper visual field stimuli. Neuromagnetic recordings. *Exp Brain Res* 1999; **124**(3): 287–294.

127. Wang L, Barber C, Kakigi R, Kaneoke Y, Okusa T, Wen Y. A first comparison of the human multifocal visual evoked magnetic field and visual evoked potential. *Neurosci Lett* 2001; **315**(1–2): 13–16.

128. Hatanaka K, Nakasato N, Seki K, Mizoi K, Yoshimoto T. Striate cortical generators of the N75, P100 and N145 components localized by pattern reversal visual evoked magnetic fields. *Tohoku J Exp Med* 1997; **182**: 9–14.

129. Shigeto H, Tobimatsu S, Yamamoto T, Kobayashi T, Kato M. Visual evoked cortical magnetic responses to checkerboard pattern reversal stimulation: a study on the neural generators of N75, P100 and N145. *J Neurol Sci* 1998; **156**(2): 186–194.

130. Hashimoto T, Kashii S, Kikuchi M, Honda Y, Nagamine T, Shibasaki H. Temporal profile of visual evoked responses to pattern-reversal stimulation analyzed with a whole-head magnetometer. *Exp Brain Res* 1999; **125**(3): 375–382.

131. Nakamura M, Kakigi R, Okusa T, Hoshiyama M, Watanabe K. Effects of check size on pattern reversal visual evoked magnetic field and potential. *Brain Res* 2000; **872**(2): 77–86.

132. Barnikol UB, Amunts K, Dammers J, *et al.* Pattern reversal visual evoked responses of V1/V2 and V5/MT as revealed by MEG combined with probabilistic cytoarchitectonic maps. *NeuroIimage* 2006; **31**(1): 86–108.

133. Inoue T, Fujimura M, Kumabe T, Nakasato N, Higano S, Tominaga T. Combined three-dimensional anisotropy contrast imaging and magnetoencephalography guidance to preserve visual function in a patient with an occipital lobe tumor. *Minim Invasive Neurosurg* 2004; **47**(4): 249–252.

134. Nakasato N, Seki K, Fujita S, *et al.* Clinical application of visual evoked fields using an MRI-linked whole head MEG system. *Front Med Biol Eng* 1996; **7**(4): 275–283.

135. Armstrong RA, Slaven A, Harding GF. Visual evoked magnetic fields to flash and pattern in 100 normal subjects. *Vision Res* 1991; **31**(11): 1859–1864.

136. Grover KM, Bowyer SM, Rock J, *et al.* Retrospective review of MEG visual evoked hemifield responses prior to resection of temporo-parieto-occipital lesions. *J Neurooncol* 2006; **77**: 161–166.

137. Anderson SJ, Holliday IE, Harding GF. Assessment of cortical dysfunction in human strabismic amblyopia using magnetoencephalography (MEG). *Vision Res* 1999; **39**(9): 1723–1738.

138. Suzuki K, Okuda J, Nakasato N, *et al.* Spatio-temporal pattern of visual evoked magnetic fields in patients with cerebral infarction in the left medial occipital lobe. In: Yoshimoto T, Kotani M, Kuriki S, Karibe H, Nakasato N, eds. *Recent Advances in Biomagnetism.* Sendai: Tohoku University Press. 1999; 708–711.

139. Hatanaka K, Nakasato N, Nagamatsu K, *et al.* Modification of the pattern-evoked magnetic fields associated with the location of the lesion along the visual pathways. In: Nenonen J, Ilmoniemi RJ, Katila T, eds. *Biomag, 2000: Proceedings of the*

12th International Conference on Biomagnetism; 2000 Aug 13–17; Espoo, Finland. Helsinki, Helsinki Univ. Technology; 2001, 145–149.

140. Ohde H, Shinoda K, Nishiyama T, *et al*. New method for detecting misrouted retinofugal fibers in humans with albinism by magnetoencephalography. *Vision Res* 2004; **44**(10): 1033–1038.

141. Lauronen L, Jalkanen R, Huttunen J, *et al*. Abnormal crossing of the optic fibres shown by evoked magnetic fields in patients with ocular albinism with a novel mutation in the OA1 gene. *Br J Ophthalmol* 2005; **89**(7): 820–824.

142. Papanicolaou AC, Simos PG, Breier JI, *et al*. Magnetoencephalographic mapping of the language specific cortex. *J Neurosurg* 1999; **90**(1): 85–93.

143. Breier JI, Simos PG, Zouridakis G, Papanicolaou AC. Lateralization of activity associated with language function using magnetoencephalography: a reliability study. *J Clin Neurophysiol* 2000; **17**(5): 503–510.

144. Lee D, Sawrie SM, Simos PG, Killen J, Knowlton RC. Reliability of language mapping with magnetic source imaging in epilepsy surgery candidates. *Epilepsy Behav* 2006; **8**(4): 742–749.

145. Breier JI, Simos PG, Zouridakis G, *et al*. Language dominance determined by magnetic source imaging: a comparison with the Wada procedure. *Neurology* 1999; **53**: 938–945.

146. Szymanski MD, Perry DW, Gage NM, *et al*. Magnetic source imaging of late evoked field responses to vowels: toward an assessment of hemispheric dominance for language. *J Neurosurg* 2001; **94**(3): 445–453.

147. Maestú F, Ortiz T, Fernandez A, *et al*. Spanish language mapping uing MEG: a validation study. *NeuroImage* 2002; **17**(3): 1579–1586.

148. Bowyer SM, Moran JE, Weiland BJ, *et al*. Language laterality determined by MEG mapping with MR-FOCUSS. *Epilepsy Behav* 2005; **6**: 235–241.

149. Kamada K, Takeuchi F, Kuriki S, Todo T, Morita A, Sawamura Y. Expressive and receptive language areas determined by a non-invasive reliable method using functional magnetic resonance imaging and magnetoencephalography. *Neurosurgery* 2007; **60**(2): 296–305.

150. Simos PG, Breier JI, Maggio WW, *et al*. Atypical temporal lobe language representation: MEG and intraoperative stimulation mapping correlation. *Neuroreport* 1999; **10**(1): 139–142.

151. Simos PG, Papanicolaou AC, Breier JI, *et al*. Localization of language-specific cortex by using magnetic source imaging and electrical stimulation mapping. *J Neurosurg* 1999; **91**(5): 787–796.

152. Castillo EM, Simos PG, Venkataraman V, Breier JI, Wheless JW, Papanicolaou AC. Mapping of expressive language cortex using magnetic source imaging. *Neurocase* 2001; **7**(5): 419–422.

153. Bowyer SM, Fleming T, Greenwald ML, *et al*. MEG localization of the basal temporal language area. *Epilepsy Behav* 2005; **6**: 229–234.

154. Grummich P, Nimsky C, Pauli E, Buchfelder M, Ganslandt O. Combining fMRI and MEG increases the reliability of presurgical language localization: a clinical study on the difference between and congruence of both modalities. *NeuroImage* 2006; **32**(4):1793–1803.

155. Simos PG, Papanicolaou AC, Breier JI, *et al.* Insights into brain function and neural plasticity using magnetic source imaging. *J Clin Neurophysiol* 2000; **17**(2): 143–162.

156. Maestú F, Saldana C, Amo C, *et al.* Can small lesions induce language reorganization as large lesions do? *Brain Lang* 2004; **89**(3): 433–438.

157. Pataraia E, Simos PG, Castillo EM, *et al.* Reorganization of language-specific cortex in patients with lesions or mesial temporal epilepsy. *Neurology* 2004; **63**(10): 1825–1832.

158. Breier JI, Castillo EM, Simos PG, *et al.* Atypical language representation in patients with chronic seizure disorder and achievement deficits with magnetoencephalography. *Epilepsia* 2005; **46**: 540–548.

159. Papanicolaou AC, Simos PG, Castillo EM, *et al.* Magnetoencephalography: a noninvasive alternative to the Wada procedure. *J Neurosurg* 2004; **100**(5): 867–876.

160. Papanicolaou AC, Pazo-Alvarez P, Castillo EM, *et al.* Functional neuroimaging with MEG: normative language profiles. *NeuroImage* 2006; **33**(1): 326–342.

161. Sarvas, J. Basic mathematical and electromagnetic concepts of the biomagnetic inverse problem. *Phys Med Biol* 1987; **32**: 11–22.

162. Merrifield WS, Simos PG, Papanicolaou AC, Philpott LM, Sutherling WW. Hemispheric language dominance in magnetoencephalography: sensitivity, specificity, and data reduction techniques. *Epilepsy Behav* 2007; **10**(1): 120–128.

163. Simos PG, Sarkari S, Castillo EM, *et al.* Reproducibility of measures of neurophysiological activity in Wernicke's area: a magnetic source imaging study. *Clin Neurophysiol* 2005; **116**(10): 2381–2391.

164. Bowyer SM, Moran JE, Mason KM, *et al.* MEG localization of language specific cortex utilizing MR-FOCUSS. *Neurology* 2004; **62**: 2247–2255.

165. Hirata M, Kato A, Taniguchi M, *et al.* Determination of language dominance with synthetic aperture magnetometry: comparison with the Wada test. *NeuroImage* 2004; **23**(1): 46–53.

166. Pataraia E, Billingsley-Marshall RL, Castillo EM, *et al.* Organization of receptive language-specific cortex before and after left temporal lobectomy. *Neurology* 2005; **64**(3): 481–487.

167. Breier JI, Castillo EM, Boake C, *et al.* Spatiotemporal patterns of language-specific brain activity in patients with chronic aphasia after stroke using magnetoencephalography, *NeuroImage* 2004; **23**: 1308–1316.

168. Breier JI, Maher LM, Schmadeke S, Hasan KM, Papanicolaou AC. Changes in language-specific brain activation after therapy for aphasia using magnetoencephalography: a case study. *Neurocase* 2007; **13**: 169–177.

169. Pfurtscheller G, Aranibar A. Evaluation of event-related desynchronization (ERD) preceding and following voluntary self-paced movement. *Electroencephalogr Clin Neurophysiol* 1979; **46**(2): 138–146.

170. Klimesch W. EEG alpha and theta oscillations reflect cognitive and memory performance: a review and analysis. *Brain Res Rev* 1999; **29**(2–3): 169–195.

171. Pfurtscheller G, Lopes da Silva FH. Event-related EEG/MEG synchronization and desynchronization: basic principles. *Clin Neurophysiol* 1999; **110**(11): 1842–1857.

172. Hari R, Salmelin R, Mäkelä JP, Salenius S, Helle M. Magnetoencephalographic cortical rhythms. *Int J Psychophysiol* 1997; **26**(1–3): 51–62.

173. Kaminski MJ, Blinowska KJ. A new method of the description of the information flow in the brain structures. *Biol Cybern* 1991; **65**:203–210.

174. Kaminski M, Blinowska K, Szclenberger W. Topographic analysis of coherence and propagation of EEG activity during sleep and wakefulness. *Electroencephalogr Clin Neurophysiol* 1997; **102**: 216–227.

Postscript: Future applications of clinical MEG

Contributors

R. E. Frye

R. Rezaie

A. C. Papanicolaou

F. Maestú

A. Fernandez

C. J. Aine

S. M. Bowyer

H. Eswaran

R. T. Wakai

Overview

The focus of this handbook thus far has been to provide a procedural account of the technique of MEG/MSI, but in this postscript we address the potential future applications of clinical MEG. We review the potential utility of MEG/MSI as an adjunct to established clinical procedures used to diagnose – as well as predict – certain pathological states. This review summarizes research that has employed MEG/MSI to determine the neurophysiological profile of various disorders on the basis of recordings of spontaneous activity and/or activation recorded during sensorimotor and cognitive tasks.

First, we will review the applications of MEG in identifying normal age-related changes in cognition and acknowledge studies that have sought to characterize neurodegenerative disorders on the basis of patterns of abnormal MEG activity. Second, we assess the role of MEG in complementing the clinical profile of neurodevelopmental disorders and discuss the advent of more novel recording techniques for assessing fetal brain activity. Third, we review the contribution of MEG/MSI in distinguishing individuals with various psychiatric and neurological disorders. Finally, we comment on the efficacy of MEG/MSI in evaluating functional reorganization of the brain following cerebral insult, including its ability to predict clinical outcomes.

Normal aging and neurodegenerative disorders

Age-dependent changes in cognition

Characterizing the neural basis of normal age-dependent changes in cognition can have important clinical implications, particularly in the case of neurodegenerative disorders where a decline in cognitive function may have prognostic value. In recent years, the application of MEG to investigate age-related changes in the profile of cognitive processing among neurologically intact individuals across the lifespan has increased. For example, a study by Kovacevic and colleagues employing the auditory oddball paradigm found that the amplitude of the early M50 component increased in elderly relative to young controls [1]. This finding led the authors to suggest that the capacity to inhibit repetitive auditory stimuli diminishes as a function of age. Furthermore, this study also found the peak onset of the late activity evoked by rare tones, corresponding to the P300 event-related complex, also increased with age. Aine and coworkers replicated this age-dependent increase in the amplitude of the M50 component in the context of an auditory incidental verbal-learning task and noted a similar effect for later components ranging from ~100 to ~800 ms [2]. These results suggested that potential age-related deficits of inhibition may also be manifest in late components related to higher cognitive functions. A subsequent study by Aine and associates further examined the effects of normal aging on cognition during the visual delayed-match-to-sample paradigm and found that although the latency and amplitude of the M100 and M300 peaks were different between young and elderly controls, they were not related to differences in behavioral performance [3]. The authors concluded that these evoked-response components might reflect the use of different cognitive strategies by the young and elderly during episodic memory processing. Localization of the activation sources underlying these components further suggested differential recruitment of association regions by the two cohorts: young adults appear to rely on posterior brain regions, while elderly appear to rely on dorsolateral, prefrontal, and supramarginal regions for performing this task. Finally, correlations between MEG measures and neuropsychological test results indicated that the elderly relied more on verbal strategies to perform this visual task while the young used primarily a visual–perceptual strategy.

Alzheimer's disease and mild cognitive impairment

Potential applications of MEG include the characterization of the neural substrates of Alzheimer's disease (AD) and other conditions such as mild cognitive impairment (MCI). An increasing number of MEG researchers have used recordings of spontaneous MEG activity – and, to some extent, event-related activation – to differentiate between normal aging and the dementias. Fernandez and colleagues recorded abnormal spontaneous brain activity in individuals with AD and MCI and reported finding a prevalence of rhythmic neuromagnetic signals in low-frequency delta and theta bands in patients with dementia [4–7]. This group's initial study found an increase in slow-wave activity sources bilaterally within the temporoparietal cortices, as well as correlations between cognitive performance and temporoparietal slow-wave activity in individuals with AD [4]. In addition to replicating their earlier finding of bilaterally increased slow-wave activity, their subsequent paper reported a correlation between left hippocampal volume and increased delta and theta activity in the left temporoparietal and temporal regions [5]. Importantly, this investigation also highlighted the diagnostic utility of MEG/MSI as an adjunct to other imaging modalities: the study showed that a linear combination of left hippocampal volume and temporal theta sources correctly classified 87.1% of participants as either patients with AD or control subjects [5]. Subsequently, the Fernandez group further enhanced the potential diagnostic contribution of MEG by demonstrating that a combination of proton magnetic resonance spectroscopy (^{1}H MRS), metabolic rates (using N-acetyl-aspartate/myo-inositol; NAA/MI), and low-frequency MEG activity classified AD patients and controls with a 90% sensitivity and a 100% specificity [6]. Their more recent study also demonstrated that resting delta activity in the left parietal cortex can reliably differentiate between AD and MCI patients and predict the risk of AD for patients with MCI [7]. After a two-year follow-up, the authors calculated the relative risk to these patients for MCI's conversion to AD and estimated an increased risk of 350% in MCI patients with the highest amount of left parietal delta activity relative to MCI patients with the lowest amount [7].

In addition to the resting MEG frequency profile, event-related MEG/MSI has been used to differentiate AD patients from normal control subjects. Pekkonen and coworkers found signs of impaired processing of the early stages of audition in AD patients, who showed longer P50 and M100 latencies in the vicinity of the auditory cortex ipsilateral to the stimulated ear [8, 9]. In a series of memory studies, Maestú and colleagues showed the usefulness of MEG/MSI for differentiating between normal aging and AD [10–12]. Specifically, they found that patients with AD exhibited a reduction in the number of late component sources (∼400 to 700 ms) in the left temporoparietal cortices during a working memory task but an increase in the number of these sources in the prefrontal cortical regions [10]. This study also demonstrated the clinical utility of MEG/MSI by showing that the number of activation sources in the left temporoparietal region significantly correlated with behavioral measures of cognitive performance and daily function. In a second study using a probe-letter memory task, these authors reported a significant correlation between late component sources predominantly in the left temporal lobe, and hippocampal volume, which indicated that degree of atrophy in mesial temporal structures was related to a reduction in the number of late component sources in the left temporal cortex [11]. Maestú and colleagues then compared activation pro-files, acquired during a memory task, with the MR spectroscopy [12]. Thus a region of interest for biochemical analysis was established for the parietotem-poral cortex, where a lower number of dipoles were found in previous studies in AD patients. Linear regression analysis revealed a high negative correlation between MEG and spectroscopy data in that the higher values of the NAA/MI ratio correlated with the lower number of activity sources between 400 and 800 ms over the parietotemporal regions. Additionally, the higher the NAA/MI ratio and the lower the number of activity sources over the parietotemporal regions between 400 and 800 ms predicted the patients' scores on cognitive and functional scales [12].

Abnormal evoked-response profiles have also been demonstrated in patients with MCI. A study by Puregger and coworkers found that, relative to controls, patients with MCI tended to exhibit increased activity associated with encoding over left frontal and temporal areas in response to nonsemantic compared to semantic words [13]. Based on this finding, the authors suggested that pro-gressive neurodegeneration may engage compensatory neural mechanisms for semantic processing in these individuals. In their study, Maestú and colleagues employed a modified version of the Sternberg task to demonstrate that, dur-ing the presentation of both target and nontarget stimuli, patients with MCI, in contrast to controls, exhibited bilateral increases in activity of the "ventral pathway" (and the ventral prefrontal cortex, middle temporal gyrus, and medial temporal lobe) [14]. Since no differences in behavioral measures were found between the two groups, the authors suggested the possibility that MCI patients may require the recruitment of additional neural networks to achieve a normal level of cognitive performance.

Parkinson's disease and Lewy body dementia

MEG may also contribute to differential diagnosis of Parkinson's disease (PD) and Lewy body dementia (LBD). Abnormal resting-state oscillatory activity has been observed in PD. For example, Kotini and coworkers reported a dif-fuse pattern of slow waves in a small sample of patients [15]. Bosboom and colleagues were able to distinguish nondemented PD patients from those mani-festing dementia symptoms [16]. Their study attempted to differentiate between different stages of PD by demonstrating that a widespread increase in theta and a decrease in beta power was concomitant with a focal decrease in gamma power in the central parietal region. Those manifesting dementia exhibited a greater increase in delta power and a decrease in relative alpha power. Stoffers and coworkers [17] elaborated on these findings with a larger systematic study. They reported that while the profile of oscillatory activity in nondemented PD patients was characterized by a diffuse increase in theta and a low alpha power over all areas except the frontal regions with decreases in posterior beta and cen-troparietal gamma power, nondemented patients exhibited increases in theta power in the left frontal, right parietal, and both central regions, in addition to decreases in widespread beta and frontal gamma power. Furthermore, these authors also noted that the changes in spectral power in PD patients were independent of disease severity, stage, and duration [17].

The possible contributions of MEG to Lewy Body Dementia (LBD) has been explored in one study by Franciotti and coworkers [18], who found that, compared to controls, patients with severe AD and LBD exhibited a significant loss of coherence in the alpha band that was more pronounced in the left hemisphere for the AD patients and in the right hemisphere in LBD. The authors suggest that these findings would ostensibly be related to the distinct cognitive disturbances characteristic of each condition.

Neurodevelopmental disorders

Fetal MEG

One of the most novel applications of MEG has been the imaging of fetal cortical activity. The possibility of characterizing anomalies in neural function early in gestation may aid in the early detection of abnormal development. Advances in multichannel SQUID design have led to the development of sophisticated techniques capable of measuring brain function *in utero* while isolating myogenic artifacts emanating from the fetal and maternal heart, as well as the uterus [19–21]. Though small in number, several studies have hinted at the potential for recording both evoked and spontaneous fetal MEG. The main finding in fetal MEG studies to date has been the successful recording of the auditory evoked response, first accomplished by Blum and colleagues in 1985 using a single-channel recording unit [22]. Over the course of several studies, other researchers, using pure tone stimulation, have characterized the fetal analogue to the M100 auditory evoked-response component as occurring at latencies ranging from ~125 to ~200 ms and amplitudes ranging from ~30 to ~175 fT [21, 23–26]. Other investigators measured the fetal auditory evoked field but reported different latency ranges [27–29]. Though not as stable as auditory, visual evoked responses also have been recorded in fetuses. Fetal visual evoked responses peaked at ~200 ms in about 58% of fetuses as early as the third trimester of pregnancy (28 weeks) and decreased (poststimulus) with an increase in gestational age [30, 31]. Furthermore, spontaneous fetal activity recorded by Eswaran and colleagues showed evidence of the process of maturation similar to EEG results for preterm babies born within the third trimester [32].

Dyslexia

Different groups of researchers have explored the possibility of deriving activation profiles characteristic of dyslexic children and adults. In a series of systematic studies, Simos and colleagues consistently demonstrated that the pattern of activation for dyslexic children during reading differs markedly from that of normal readers [33–38]. Patterns for dyslexic children indicate reduced activation of the left posterior superior temporal/supramarginal gyri – primarily the posterior superior temporal region – accompanied by hyperactivation of the right homotopic regions, a compensatory increase in prefrontal activity, and a marked delay in the onset of activity within temporoparietal regions, mainly in the left superior temporal gyrus. Interestingly, as pointed out by Papanicolaou and coworkers [37], the same dyslexic children exhibit a normal pattern of left hemispheric dominance for aural receptive language, thus refuting the long-standing hypothesis [39] that the disorder is related to anomalous hemispheric dominance for language at large.

MEG/MSI has also been used to address the notion that individuals with dyslexia possess deficits in perceiving the basic units of speech, presumably due to an inability to process rapidly changing auditory information. For example, Nagarajan and associates reported that after being presented with successive, rapid, pure tones, dyslexic adults exhibited a significant reduction of M100 auditory evoked field, as well as weaker beta and gamma band coherence, relative to nonimpaired adults [40]. These findings were supported by Renvall and Hari who found that, compared to controls, dyslexic adults exhibited a weaker bilateral M100 response during an acoustic transition from noise to square-wave stimuli that simulated a fricative consonant to a vowel transition [41]. Examining more complex constituents of auditory linguistic stimuli, Helenius and coworkers exposed dyslexic and nonimpaired adults to natural bisyllabic and monosyllabic stimuli and to pairs of complex nonspeech sounds or tones [42]. They reported finding abnormally large M100 amplitudes only when the dyslexic adults responded to the natural bisyllabic and monosyllabic stimuli, but not when presented with nonspeech sounds; the response normalized when the initial formant transition (the consonant) was removed from the syllable. The authors speculated that the response difference was related to the processing of rapid frequency transitions. A similar study by Parviainen and colleagues did not replicate this difference in the amplitude of the M100 response between dyslexic and nonimpaired adults, though a relative attenuation in the latency onset of this component for syllabic stimuli was present, so that dyslexic individuals failed to demonstrate the typical earlier peak in the left compared to the right hemisphere [43]. In addition to reporting differences in amplitude and latency onset, several authors also observed aberrant lateralization of the underlying source of the M100 component when evoked by consonant–vowel syllables. Heim and associates reported greater posterior localization in the right perisylvian region in dyslexic adults relative to nonimpaired readers [44]. This deviation in asymmetry along the anterior–posterior axis was also seen during auditory syllabic processing by dyslexic children in the early auditory evoked field [45] and the later M260 component [46].

Autism spectrum disorders

Characterization of the neural phenotype of autism spectrum disorder (ASD) is one the faster growing applications of MEG. To date, several investigators have attempted to distinguish the neurophysiological profile of ASD from that of normal subjects on the basis of recordings of spontaneous brain activity and, to a larger extent, on the basis of evoked responses during execution of cognitive functions potentially underlying deficits representative of the disorder. While studies of spontaneous recordings among individuals with ASD are few, they have hinted at the possibility that the underlying pathology of the disorder may in some cases be neurophysiological activity similar to that of specific epileptic conditions. For example, an early investigation by Lewine and coworkers found that children with regressive-type autism showed evidence of epileptiform activity during stage III sleep localized to the left perisylvian region, similar to children with classic Landau–Kleffner syndrome [47]. The authors also noted that a majority of the autistic children studied exhibited a multifocal profile of abnormal spontaneous activity with spike-wave discharges localized to the right perisylvian and frontal regions. In a study of children with early-onset ASD, Muñoz-Yunta and colleagues [48] also localized epileptiform discharges in the perisylvian regions in a similar proportion of subjects as those reported in the Lewine study. These authors also emphasized the diagnostic utility of MEG for differentiating patients with autism from those with Asperger's syndrome in that the latter group manifested more epileptic discharges in the right perisylvian cortex, while the former exhibited a bilateral distribution of epileptiform activity sources, with a slight leftward preponderance.

Studies of evoked MEG activity in ASD have largely focused on establishing profiles of aberrant auditory processing, particularly in relation to developmental language impairments that may underlie disabilities in communication which are characteristic of the individuals diagnosed with ASD. Gage and colleagues [49] proposed an abnormal maturational trajectory of the auditory system based on their findings that children with ASD exhibited bilateral prolongation of the M100 latency accompanied by an age-related increase in the onset of this component in the right hemisphere. The ASD pattern is opposite to the linear decrease in this latency with age typically seen in normally developing children. The authors corroborated their previous finding in another study [50] in which they found a reduction in the dynamic frequency range of the M100 component in the right hemisphere. They suggested that this asymmetry may be related to diminished neural conduction rates in the auditory cortex critical to frequency encoding. The concept of an abnormal course of maturation in ASD was supported in a subsequent study by Flagg and coworkers who reported that the lateralization of late-onset components evoked by passive auditory presentation of vowels was opposite in normal and autistic children [51]. Whereas in typically developing children the component became increasingly leftwardly asymmetric as a function of age, children with ASD exhibited a profile of progressively greater right-hemisphere dominance with increased age. Anomalous lateralization of the auditory evoked response in children and adolescents with autism also was observed by Wilson and colleagues [52], such that the left-hemisphere gamma oscillatory activity in the ~200 to ~500 ms latency range was reduced in power. This reduction indicated a lack of coherent interactions between cortical neurons in the left primary auditory cortex.

Roberts and coworkers [53] also cited current work by their group [54, 55] that showed anomalies in the anterioposterior shift of the M100 component in the right hemisphere of children with ASD, similar to the shift seen in children with dyslexia [45] and correlated with neurophysiological measures of fundamental linguistic skills. A deviation from the normal profile of localization of this component may be related to impaired language function in ASD children.

Oram Cardy and colleagues [56] reported that the magnetic mismatch field, in response to either syllables or acoustically matched tones, in autistic children was delayed by ~50 ms relative to typically developing children. Based on this finding, the authors suggested that detection of syllables may be retarded and result in impaired processing of continuous streams of syllables. In a concurrent study of rapid temporal processing in those with impaired auditory speech perception [57], these authors presented pair tones separated by variable intervals to children with ASD, to those with specific language impairment, and to controls. They found that, while no differences in the auditory evoked fields were discernible for longer intervals (800 ms), the M50 and M100 components evoked by the second tone at the shorter interval (150 ms) were absent in children with autism and specific language impairment. Since children with Asperger's syndrome without language deficits exhibited a profile similar to that of controls, the authors suggested that language impairment may reflect a specific phenotype within the autistic spectrum.

Attention deficit hyperactivity disorder (ADHD)

The few MEG studies conducted thus far provide some insights into the neurophysiological activity profile underlying ADHD and may potentially have some diagnostic value in the future. For example, using an adaptation of the Wisconsin Card Sorting Task in an exploratory study [58], Mulas and colleagues found that while normal children exhibited a spatiotemporal profile of late-onset activity sources that progressed from the medial temporal to anterior cingulate cortex when evoked by set-shifting cues, children with ADHD showed activation of the inferior parietal and posterior superior temporal cortices. To a degree, the findings from this study indicate the neurological underpinnings of executive dysfunction prevalent in children with ADHD [59, 60].

In a more recent study, Dockstader and coworkers reported that following random median-nerve stimulation, adults with ADHD demonstrated weaker rebound of beta activity in the primary and secondary cortices relative to normal adults [61]. These findings, the authors speculated, may explain in part deficits in sensory feedback previously noted in subjects with ADHD or, alternatively, may reflect the top-down influence of impaired attention on somatosensory processing in these individuals.

Epileptic aphasia

Children with epilepsy manifesting aphasic symptoms represent a rare subgroup of neurodevelopmental disorders. An MEG study by Lewine and colleagues found that children with classic Landau–Kleffner syndrome exhibited epileptiform activity limited to the left perisylvian region during stage III sleep, which relates to the progressive aphasia that is a hallmark of these individuals [47]. Subsequently, Wolff and coworkers reported that in children with benign partial epilepsy, those exhibiting focal discharges in left perisylvian regions were most severely impaired on tests of language function [62]. Castillo and colleagues explored the utility of MEG in the diagnosis of epileptic aphasia by investigating two children with Landau–Kleffner syndrome [63]. The study showed that while one patient exhibited clear linguistic regression, the other showed progressive improvement of function, though recordings of spontaneous activity revealed focal epileptiform discharges in the left perisylvian cortex in both cases. Sources of evoked responses obtained in the context of an auditory word-recognition task were found within the same areas where the epileptiform discharges originated in the patient with severe language dysfunction, but in homotopic regions of the unaffected (right) perisylvian cortex in the patient with improved linguistic function. Incidentally, a 2-year follow-up of the impaired patient following multiple subpial transections not only showed an absence of epileptiform discharges but also indicated increased language-related activation in the left perisylvian cortex during the same word comprehension task.

Psychiatric disorders

Schizophrenia

Early applications of whole-head MEG revealed the presence of increased slow-wave activity in temporoparietal regions among small samples of patients with schizophrenia [64–66]. Over the course of several systematic studies [67–70], investigators also used MEG and substantially larger sample sizes to verify the incidence of abnormally high slow-wave activity in patients with schizophrenia in contrast to nonpsychotic individuals. Fehr and coworkers [67] reported that relative to nonpsychotic controls, patients with schizophrenia exhibited enhanced delta and theta band activity localized in posterior and frontotemporal regions. Importantly, this study also revealed that positive symptom scores varied as a function of delta and theta activity in the frontal regions, a finding that suggested that focal abnormal slow-wave activity may be a defining feature of schizophrenia. In another sample of schizophrenic patients [68], these authors reported observing focal increases in delta and theta activity within the parietal and temporal areas, with slow waves in the latter region significantly correlating to negative symptoms. The potential diagnostic value of slow-wave localization was further highlighted by Wienbruch and coworkers [69]. They also found elevated delta and theta activity in temporal and parietal regions in schizophrenic patients that significantly correlated with measures of auditory hallucinations and differentiated these patients from individuals with major depression. More recently, these findings were replicated by Rockstroh and associates, who further stressed the diagnostic potential of MEG in psychosis [70].

In addition to studies of spontaneous slow-wave activity, the diagnostic potential of MEG has been explored in sensory activation studies addressing the hypothesis that schizophrenia may be associated with abnormal hemispheric specialization [71, 72]. In a series of studies, Reite and colleagues tested this hypothesis by mapping the sources of the M100 auditory evoked response [73–77] and of the somatosensory M20 [78] and M50 [79] evoked-response components in patients with schizophrenia and in nonpsychotic controls. Data from the studies of the auditory responses have showed aberrant hemispheric differences in the localization of the sources of the M100 component in patients with schizophrenia. The hemispheric differences in source localization varied as a function of gender and was reminiscent of the well-known gender differences in the age of onset in schizophrenia [80]. The aberrant pattern of source localization of the M100 component in patients with schizophrenia has been confirmed by other investigators [81–83]. Tiihonen and coworkers [83] also reported a relationship between the degree of aberration in source of localization and the severity of schizophrenic symptoms. With respect to somatosensory evoked fields, early support for the hypothesis that schizophrenia is associated with abnormal cerebral lateralization was provided by Reite and coworkers who found reversed lateral asymmetry in the locus of the M20 component sources in patients relative to nonpsychotic individuals [78]. More recently, the same authors confirmed their earlier results by reporting a similar pattern for the M50 somatosensory component sources [79].

Depression

On the basis of the frequency content of spontaneous brain activity, Wienbruch and colleagues differentiated patients with schizophrenia and normal controls from patients diagnosed with major depression by noting a significant reduction in delta and theta activity in the frontal/prefrontal regions in the latter group [69]. These authors also reported a significant relationship between slow-wave activity in the frontal/prefrontal regions and depression scale scores. Their findings led the authors to suggest a relationship between symptom severity and reduction of anterior slow-wave activity in major depressive disorder. Similarly, Rockstroh and coworkers reported an identical finding of reduced anterior delta and theta activity accompanied by a trend for increased slow-wave activity in parieto-occipital regions that correlated with the clinical symptoms of patients with major depression [70]. Indeed, the tendency for increased slow-wave activity in posterior brain regions noted by these authors [70] is in line with an earlier systematic study of major depressive disorder by Fernandez and colleagues [84] who found increased delta activity – also associated with symptom severity – in the occipital lobe to be a reliable risk factor for depression. In addition to increases in slow-wave activity, patients with major depressive disorder also exhibit aberrant steady-state visual evoked field (ssVEF) profiles, as reported by Moratti and colleagues [85]. These aberrant ssVEF profiles are related to neuropsychological models of depression based on low emotional arousal. Specifically, these authors found that relative to controls, females with clinical depression exhibited reduced activation in the right temporoparietal cortex, marked by a reduction in the amplitude of the ssVEF in response to high-arousing emotional stimuli.

Obsessive-compulsive disorder (OCD)

In a preliminary MEG study of patients with OCD, Amo and coworkers reported prevalent frontotemporal paroxysmal rhythmic discharges originating mainly in limbic regions [86]. The authors hypothesized that the condition may be attributable to a dysfunction on the corticostriatal network. More recently, Maihöfner and colleagues proposed an alternative explanation to the pathogenesis of the disorder based on their findings of increased beta activity in the left superior temporal gyrus accompanied by elevated activity in the delta/theta band within the left dorsolateral prefrontal cortex of patients with OCD relative to controls [87].

Post-traumatic stress disorder (PTSD)

In the context of anxiety disorders, a few MEG studies have sought to characterize patients with PTSD on the basis of profiles of abnormal slow-wave oscillatory activity. An initial study of individuals with PTSD by Ray and coworkers found a positive correlation between focal delta activity sources in the left ventro-lateral frontal cortex and the number of dissociative experiences [88]. These authors hypothesized that the increased focal slow-wave activity in individuals with PTSD may reflect decoupling of frontal circuits involved in emotion from left hemisphere language regions, supporting the conjecture that dissociative experiences are characterized by disrupted access to structured verbal memory related to traumatic events. In a large-scale systematic study Kolassa and associates observed increased delta activity in the left insula with accompanying right hemisphere prefrontal slow-wave sources in patients with PTSD relative to controls [89]. Accordingly, these authors speculated that the findings in the insular cortex may be related to symptoms of alexithymia previously reported in PTSD, whereas the abnormal oscillatory activity in the frontal region may lead to diminished fear extinction and reduced inhibition of limbic structures.

Neurological disorders

Tinnitus

Among the neurological disorders which MEG has been used to address is tinnitus. An early MEG study of tinnitus by Hoke and coworkers [90] used tonal stimulation to characterize the condition and demonstrated that the amplitude ratio of the M200/M100 components in these patients was abnormally small due to an augmented M100 response, though subsequent investigators were unable to replicate this finding using similar approaches [91, 92]. Abnormal modulation of these components has also been found during artificial inducement of tinnitus in normal controls using discotheque music. Emmerich and coworkers observed a transient delay and prolongation of the M100 component along with decreased conspicuity of the other auditory evoked field waveforms – including the M200 – in individuals exposed to musical stimulation relative to those unexposed [93].

In addition to differences in the amplitude of the classic auditory evoked field components, other researchers have approached the study of tinnitus through tonotopic mapping in the auditory cortex of these patients. Muhlnickel and coworkers found that the sources of auditory responses evoked by tones in the tinnitus frequency in patients were significantly shifted relative to source generators evoked by corresponding frequencies in neurologically intact controls [94]. In addition, they found a strong association between the extent of cortical source shift and subjective strength of the tinnitus, suggesting that the condition may be characterized by abnormal neural plasticity of the auditory cortex. Applying the 40 Hz auditory steady-state response paradigm and using different carrier frequencies (384 to 6561 Hz), Wienbruch and colleagues reported that, relative to controls, patients with chronic tinnitus exhibited bilateral shifts in the location of auditory response sources within the primary auditory cortex [95].

Additional studies of patients with tinnitus have explored the possibility of abnormalities in spontaneous neuromagnetic activity: Weisz and coworkers found that patients with tinnitus exhibited a reduction in alpha and accompanying increase in delta activity over the temporal lobe regions compared to control participants [96]. The activity changes were strongly associated with the level of tinnitus-related stress reported by these patients. A subsequent study by these authors demonstrated that following a period of steady slow-wave activity, patients with tinnitus exhibited an increase in gamma-band activity relative to controls [97]. More recently, Bowyer and colleagues addressed the utility of spontaneous MEG for identifying tinnitus [98]. They used a coherence analysis and found that in patients with tinnitus, high magnitudes of coherent activity in the auditory cortex contralateral to the patients' perceived tinnitus was consistently present, in contrast to control subjects who showed no intraregional coherence among multiple foci of activity.

Tremor syndromes

While dementia is a prominent feature of the neurodegenerative process in a significant number of patients with Parkinson's disease (PD), these patients are also afflicted by notable degradation of motor functions characterized by tremors. However, this symptom of PD may also be manifest in other tremor syndromes with different etiologies. Timmerman and colleagues reported on the neurophysiological profile of tremor in patients with PD using measures of cerebromuscular and cerebro-cerebral coherence [99]. In general, these authors indicated that tremor-related activity in PD can be characterized by aberrant coupling in a cerebello-diencephalic-cortical loop and cortical motor (M1, SMA/CMA, PM) and sensory (SII, PPC) areas contralateral to the limb exhibiting tremors. Timmerman and coworkers subsequently applied MEG to successfully differentiate between tremor syndromes in patients with PD and patients with hepatic encephalopathy exhibiting postural tremors [100].

Multiple sclerosis (MS)

Cover and coworkers attempted to differentiate between MS patients and healthy controls on the basis of a significant decrease in interhemispheric coherence of alpha activity in MS [101]. From their findings, the authors suggested that the disorder may arise from aberrant long-range connectivity. A subsequent study by Kotini and colleagues found that relative to controls, patients with MS exhibited a diffuse abnormal rhythmic activity pattern characterized by lower amplitude and frequencies within the 2 to 7 Hz range [102]. Using complex mathematical modeling techniques, Georgopoulos and colleagues are developing procedures for classifying individual subjects into various patient groups, including MS, based on measures of spontaneous neuromagnetic activity [103].

Brain tumors

Though MEG serves an important purpose in the evaluation of patients with brain tumors in the context of presurgical functional mapping, recordings of spontaneous neuromagnetic activity in tumor patients may also facilitate assessment of the extent of pathology. For example, de Jongh and colleagues were the first to characterize the effects of glioma on the integrity of surrounding tissue using recordings of spontaneous MEG [104]. They demonstrated that sources of delta and theta activity were localized in the vicinity of the tumor in contrast to gamma activity sources that were located in the contralateral hemisphere. Kamada and coworkers reported increases in slow-wave activity around tumors in 4 of 7 patients [105]. The diagnostic utility of MEG was further demonstrated in a later study by Baayen and associates that showed localization of the sources of abnormal low-frequency activity around tumors in 13 of 20 patients with clinical seizures associated with these tumors [106]. Oshino and colleagues also found increased intensity of delta and theta activity in the tissue adjacent to the tumor, as well as in the area of edema surrounding the tumors, in 13 of 15 patients studied [107]. Several authors also reported on the relationship between abnormal low-frequency MEG activity and tumor characteristics. de Jongh's group found that more malignant and larger tumors were associated with higher delta power [108], and Oshino and associates demonstrated that delta power was greater for intra-axial tumors involving subcortical fibers than for extra-axial tumors [107].

Cerebral ischemia and stroke

Changes in spontaneous MEG associated with acute stroke and cortical ischemia may also be important in evaluating the degree to which these forms of insult affect the integrity of the preserved tissues and their relationship to brain function and clinical outcomes. In a study of patients having suffered transient ischemic attacks, Stippich and colleagues found that delta and theta activity originating in the sensorimotor cortex provided a robust index of functional recovery for a short period after the insult [109]. Tecchio and coworkers reported that, in patients with acute stroke in one hemisphere, reduction of gamma-band activity concurrent with an increase in slow-wave power in the middle-cerebral-artery region of the affected hemisphere was related to worse clinical outcome [110]. Interestingly, this study also showed that increases in low-frequency rhythms in the perilesional tissue extended, though to a lesser degree, to homotopic regions in the unaffected hemisphere. Indeed, Seki and colleagues showed that, in patients with internal carotid artery occlusive disease, neuromagnetic sources of theta activity were also diffuse in nature reaching beyond perilesional tissue and not necessarily localizing to the region ipsilateral to the infarct [111].

A later study of patients with acute stroke by Tecchio and coworkers also showed that strength of delta activity sources increased in regions both ipsi- and contra-lateral to the infarct [112]. While this metric did not correlate with clinical status in the acute phase of stroke, a correlation did occur between delta dipole strength and clinical recovery in the postacute phase. The authors also observed that the magnitude of slow-wave activity varied as a function of the lesion. More recently, Castillo and coworkers demonstrated the relationship between abnormal slow-wave activity and impaired sensory function in postacute unilateral stroke patients [113]. They found that the reduction in amplitude of primary sensory cortex responses evoked by stimulation of the affected hand in patients with severe sensory deficits was related to the density of delta dipoles over the postcentral region.

Functional reorganization

Cerebrovascular disease

The use of MEG in documenting brain plasticity for sensorimotor functions following stroke has been demonstrated in several studies by Rossini and colleagues [112, 114, 115]. They showed the reorganization of the early M20 and M30 somatosensory evoked-response sources and explored its relationship to clinical outcomes. In an investigation of individuals recovering from stroke, Rossini and coworkers found significant alterations in the location and latency of the M20 and M30 source generators in the primary sensory hand area of the affected and, to a lesser extent, unaffected hemispheres, though more favorable outcomes were correlated with reorganization within the ipsilesional hemisphere [114]. Studies by Tecchio and coworkers have reaffirmed this earlier finding in both chronic and acute stoke patients by reporting positive correlations between reorganization of M20 and M30 cortical sources in the perirolandic region of the affected hemisphere and recovery of hand function [112, 115].

MEG has not only been used to measure cortical reorganization for sensorimotor functions but has also been applied to monitor neural plasticity related to receptive language function following recovery from stroke. In a study of individuals with chronic aphasia secondary to left-hemisphere ischemic stroke, Breier and coworkers observed that receptive language functions were predominantly reorganized to areas outside the classic Wernicke's region in the ipsilesional hemisphere as opposed to the unaffected hemisphere [116]. These authors also reported that improved clinical outcome was associated with normalization of activity in putative premorbid receptive language regions, in contrast to activity reorganized in perilesional areas outside premorbid language areas that may become involved in language after aphasia secondary to stroke. Reorganization of receptive language regions in chronic aphasic patients has been studied systematically in the context of constraint-induced language therapy [117]. The most adequate responders to therapy showed bilaterally increased activity in posterior receptive language regions. Altered MEG activity in individuals with chronic apha-sia was addressed in a post-therapy study by Meinzer and coworkers [118]. They reported on a decrease in perilesional delta activity that correlated with improved neuropsychological outcome. Their work further underlines the pre-dictive potential of MEG in the clinical assessment of patients recovering from stroke.

References

1. Kovacevic S, Qualls C, Adair JC, *et al*. Age-related effects on superior temporal gyrus activity during an auditory oddball task. *Neuroreport* 2005; **16**: 1075–1079.
2. Aine CJ, Adair JC, Knoefel JE, *et al*. Temporal dynamics of age-related differences in auditory incidental verbal learning. *Brain Res Cogn Brain Res* 2005; **24**: 1–18.
3. Aine CJ, Woodruff CC, Knoefel JE, *et al*. Aging: compensation or maturation? *NeuroImage* 2006; **32**: 1891–1904.
4. Fernandez A, Maestú F, Amo C, *et al*. Focal temporoparietal slow activity in Alzheimer's disease revealed by magnetoencephalography. *Biol Psychiatry* 2002; **52**: 764–770.
5. Fernandez A, Arrazola J, Maestú F, *et al*. Correlations of hippocampal atrophy and focal low-frequency magnetic activity in Alzheimer disease: volumetric MR imaging-magnetoencephalographic study. *AJNR Am J Neuroradiol* 2003; **24**: 481–487.
6. Fernandez A, Garcia-Segura JM, Ortiz T, *et al*. Proton magnetic resonance spectroscopy and magnetoencephalographic estimation of delta dipole density: a combination of techniques that may contribute to the diagnosis of Alzheimer's disease. *Dement Geriatr Cogn Disord* 2005; **20**: 169–177.
7. Fernandez A, Turrero A, Zuluaga P, *et al*. Magnetoencephalographic parietal delta dipole density in mild cognitive impairment: preliminary results of a method to estimate the risk of developing Alzheimer disease. *Arch Neurol* 2006; **63**: 427–430.
8. Pekkonen E, Huotilainen M, Virtanen J, Naatanen R, Ilmoniemi RJ, Erkinjuntti T. Alzheimer's disease affects parallel processing between the auditory cortices. *Neuroreport* 1996; **7**(8): 1365–1368.
9. Pekkonen E, Jaaskelainen IP, Hietanen M, *et al*. Impaired preconscious auditory processing and cognitive functions in Alzheimer's disease. *Clin Neurophysiol* 1999; **110**(11): 1942–1947.
10. Maestú F, Fernandez A, Simos PG, *et al*. Spatio-temporal patterns of brain magnetic activity during a memory task in Alzheimer's disease. *Neuroreport* 2001; **12**: 3917–3922.
11. Maestú F, Arrazola J, Fernandez A, *et al*. Do cognitive patterns of brain magnetic activity correlate with hippocampal atrophy in Alzheimer's disease? *J Neurol Neurosurg Psychiatry* 2003; **74**: 208–212.
12. Maestú F, Garcia-Segura J, Ortiz T, *et al*. Evidence of biochemical and biomagnetic interactions in Alzheimer's disease: an MEG and MR spectroscopy study. *Dement Geriatr Cogn Disord* 2005; **20**: 145–152.

13. Puregger E, Walla P, Deecke L, Dal-Bianco P. Magnetoencephalographic – features related to mild cognitive impairment. *NeuroImage* 2003; **20**: 2235–2244.
14. Maestú F, Campo P, Del Rio D, *et al.* Increased biomagnetic activity in the ventral pathway in mild cognitive impairment. *Clin Neurophysiol* 2008; **119**: 1320–1327.
15. Kotini A, Anninos P, Adamopoulos A, Prassopoulos P. Low-frequency MEG activity and MRI evaluation in Parkinson's disease. *Brain Topogr* 2005; **18**: 59–63.
16. Bosboom JL, Stoffers D, Stam CJ, *et al.* Resting state oscillatory brain dynamics in Parkinson's disease: an MEG study. *Clin Neurophysiol* 2006; **117**: 2521–2531.
17. Stoffers D, Bosboom JL, Deijen JB, Wolters EC, Berendse HW, Stam CJ. Slowing of oscillatory brain activity is a stable characteristic of Parkinson's disease without dementia. *Brain* 2007; **130**: 1847–1860.
18. Franciotti R, Iacono D, Della Penna S, *et al.* Cortical rhythms reactivity in AD, LBD and normal subjects: a quantitative MEG study. *Neurobiol Aging* 2006; **27**: 1100–1109.
19. Eswaran H, Wilson JD, Murphy P, Preissl H, Lowery CL. Application of wavelet transform to uterine electromyographic signals recorded using abdominal surface electrodes. *J Matern Fetal Neonatal Med* 2002; **11**: 158–166.
20. Vrba J, Robinson SE, McCubbin J, *et al.* Human fetal brain imaging by magnetoencephalography: verification of fetal brain signals by comparison with fetal brain models. *NeuroImage* 2004; **21**: 1009–1020.
21. Lowery CL, Eswaran H, Murphy P, Preissl H. Fetal magnetoencephalography. *Semin Fetal Neonatal Med* 2006; **11**: 430–436.
22. Blum T, Saling E, Bauer R. First magnetoencephalographic recordings of the brain activity of a human fetus. *Br J Obstet Gynaecol* 1985; **92**: 1224–1229.
23. Eswaran H, Lowery CL, Robinson SE, Wilson JD, Cheyne D, McKenzie D. Challenges of recording human fetal auditory-evoked response using magnetoencephalography. *J Matern Fetal Med* 2000; **9**: 303–307.
24. Eswaran H, Preissl H, Wilson JD, *et al.* Short-term serial magnetoencephalography recordings of fetal auditory evoked responses. *Neurosci Lett* 2002; **331**: 128–132.
25. Preissl H, Lowery CL, Eswaran H. Fetal magnetoencephalography: current progress and trends. *Exp Neurol* 2004; **190** (Suppl 1): S28–S36.
26. Holst M, Eswaran H, Lowery C, Murphy P, Norton J, Preissl H. Development of auditory evoked fields in human fetuses and newborns: a longitudinal MEG study. *Clin Neurophysiol* 2005; **116**: 1949–1955.
27. Lengle JM, Chen M, Wakai RT. Improved neuromagnetic detection of fetal and neonatal auditory evoked responses. *Clin Neurophysiol* 2001; **112**: 785–792.
28. Schneider U, Schleussner E, Haueisen J, Nowak H, Seewald HJ. Signal analysis of auditory evoked cortical fields in fetal magnetoencephalography. *Brain Topogr* 2001; **14**: 69–80.
29. Zappasodi F, Tecchio F, Pizzella V, *et al.* Detection of fetal auditory evoked responses by means of magnetoencephalography. *Brain Res* 2001; **917**: 167–173.
30. Eswaran H, Wilson J, Preissl H, *et al.* Magnetoencephalographic recordings of visual evoked brain activity in the human fetus. *Lancet* 2002; **360**: 779–780.
31. Sheridan CJ, Preissl H, Siegel ER, *et al.* Neonatal and fetal response decrement of evoked responses: a MEG study. *Clin Neurophysiol* 2008; **119**: 796–804.

32. Eswaran H, Haddad NI, Shihabuddin BS, *et al.* Non-invasive detection and identification of brain activity patterns in the developing fetus. *Clin Neurophysiol* 2007; **118**: 1940–1946.
33. Simos PG, Breier JI, Fletcher JM, Bergman E, Papanicolaou AC. Cerebral mechanisms involved in word reading in dyslexic children: a magnetic source imaging approach. *Cereb Cortex* 2000; **10**: 809–816.
34. Simos PG, Breier JI, Fletcher JM, *et al.* Brain activation profiles in dyslexic children during non-word reading: a magnetic source imaging study. *Neurosci Lett* 2000; **290**: 61–65.
35. Sarkari S, Simos PG, Fletcher JM, Castillo EM, Breier JI, Papanicolaou AC. Contributions of magnetic source imaging to the understanding of dyslexia. *Semin Pediatr Neurol* 2002; **9**: 229–238.
36. Breier JI, Simos PG, Fletcher JM, Castillo EM, Zhang W, Papanicolaou AC. Abnormal activation of temporoparietal language areas during phonetic analysis in children with dyslexia. *Neuropsychology* 2003; **17**: 610–621.
37. Papanicolaou AC, Simos PG, Breier JI, *et al.* Brain mechanisms for reading in children with and without dyslexia: a review of studies of normal development and plasticity. *Dev Neuropsychol* 2003; **24**: 593–612.
38. Simos PG, Fletcher JM, Denton C, Sarkari S, Billingsley-Marshall R, Papanicolaou AC. Magnetic source imaging studies of dyslexia interventions. *Dev Neuropsychol* 2006; **30**: 591–611.
39. Orton S. *Reading, Writing, and Speech Problems in Children*. New York: Norton, 1937.
40. Nagarajan S, Mahncke H, Salz T, Tallal P, Roberts T, Merzenich MM. Cortical auditory signal processing in poor readers. *Proc Natl Acad Sci USA* 1999; **96**: 6483–6488.
41. Renvall H, Hari R. Auditory cortical responses to speech-like stimuli in dyslexic adults. *J Cogn Neurosci* 2002; **14**: 757–768.
42. Helenius P, Salmelin R, Richardson U, Leinonen S, Lyytinen H. Abnormal auditory cortical activation in dyslexia 100 msec after speech onset. *J Cogn Neurosci* 2002; **14**: 603–617.
43. Parviainen T, Helenius P, Salmelin R. Cortical differentiation of speech and non-speech sounds at 100 ms: implications for dyslexia. *Cereb Cortex* 2005; **15**: 1054–1063.
44. Heim S, Eulitz C, Elbert T. Altered hemispheric asymmetry of auditory N100m in adults with developmental dyslexia. *Neuroreport* 2003; **14**: 501–504.
45. Heim S, Eulitz C, Elbert T. Altered hemispheric asymmetry of auditory P100m in dyslexia. *Eur J Neurosci* 2003; **17**: 1715–1722.
46. Paul I, Bott C, Heim S, Eulitz C, Elbert T. Reduced hemispheric asymmetry of the auditory N260m in dyslexia. *Neuropsychologia* 2006; **44**: 785–794.
47. Lewine JD, Andrews R, Chez M, *et al.* Magnetoencephalographic patterns of epileptiform activity in children with regressive autism spectrum disorders. *Pediatrics* 1999; **104**: 405–418.
48. Muñoz-Yunta JA, Ortiz T, Palau-Baduell M, *et al.* Magnetoencephalographic pattern of epileptiform activity in children with early-onset autism spectrum disorders. *Clin Neurophysiol* 2008; **119**: 626–634.

49. Gage NM, Siegel B, Roberts TP. Cortical auditory system maturational abnormalities in children with autism disorder: an MEG investigation. *Brain Res Dev Brain Res* 2003; **144**: 201–209.

50. Gage NM, Siegel B, Callen M, Roberts TP. Cortical sound processing in children with autism disorder: an MEG investigation. *Neuroreport* 2003; **14**: 2047–2051.

51. Flagg EJ, Cardy JE, Roberts W, Roberts TP. Language lateralization development in children with autism: insights from the late field magnetoencephalogram. *Neurosci Lett* 2005; **386**: 82–87.

52. Wilson TW, Rojas DC, Reite ML, Teale PD, Rogers SJ. Children and adolescents with autism exhibit reduced MEG steady-state gamma responses. *Biol Psychiatry* 2007; **62**: 192–197.

53. Roberts TP, Schmidt GL, Egeth M, *et al.* Electrophysiological signatures: magnetoencephalographic studies of the neural correlates of language impairment in autism spectrum disorders. *Int J Psychophysiol* 2008; **68**: 149–160.

54. Schmidt GL, Rey MM, Roberts TPL. Anatomical asymmetry of the M100 source in typically developing children and children with autism spectrum disorders. 2007; Paper presented at the Annual Meeting of the International Society for the Advancement of Clinical Magnetoencephalography, ISACM. Sendai, Japan. 2007, August 27–30.

55. Schmidt GL, Blaskey LS, Rey MM, Levy SE, Roberts TPL. Hemispheric differences in the neural correlates of rapid temporal processing in autism spectrum disorders. 2007; Abstract, Annual Meeting of the Society for Neuroscience, San Diego, CA; 2007, November.

56. Oram Cardy JE, Flagg EJ, Roberts W, Brian J, Roberts TP. Delayed mismatch field for speech and non-speech sounds in children with autism. *Neuroreport* 2005; **16**: 521–525.

57. Oram Cardy JE, Flagg EJ, Roberts W, Brian J, Roberts TP. Magnetoencephalograph identifies rapid temporal processing deficit in autism and language impairment. *Neuroreport* 2005; **16**: 329–332.

58. Mulas F, Capilla A, Fernandez S, *et al.* Shifting-related brain magnetic activity in attention-deficit/hyperactivity disorder. *Biol Psychiatry* 2006; **59**: 373–379.

59. Castellanos FX, Tannock R. Neuroscience of attention-deficit/hyperactivity disorder: the search for endophenotypes. *Nat Rev Neurosci* 2002; **3**: 617–628.

60. Boonstra AM, Oosterlaan J, Sergeant JA, Buitelaar JK. Executive functioning in adult ADHD: a meta-analytic review. *Psychol Med* 2005; **35**: 1097–1108.

61. Dockstader C, Gaetz W, Cheyne D, Wang F, Castellanos FX, Tannock R. MEG event-related desynchronization and synchronization deficits during basic somatosensory processing in individuals with ADHD. *Behav Brain Funct* 2008; **4**: 8.

62. Wolff M, Weiskopf N, Serra E, Preissl H, Birbaumer N, Kraegeloh-Mann I. Benign partial epilepsy in childhood: selective cognitive deficits are related to the location of focal spikes determined by combined EEG/MEG. *Epilepsia* 2005; **46**: 1661–1667.

63. Castillo EM, Butler IJ, Baumgartner JE, Passaro A, Papanicolaou AC. When epilepsy interferes with word comprehension: findings in Landau–Kleffner syndrome. *J Child Neurol* 2008; **23**: 97–101.

64. Cānive JM, Lewine JD, Edgar JC, *et al.* Magnetoencephalographic assessment of spontaneous brain activity in schizophrenia. *Psychopharmacol Bull* 1996; **32**: 741–750.
65. Cānive JM, Lewine JD, Edgar JC, *et al.* Spontaneous brain magnetic activity in schizophrenia patients treated with aripiprazole. *Psychopharmacol Bull* 1998; **34**: 101–105.
66. Wienbruch C. Abnormal slow wave mapping (ASWAM) – a tool for the investigation of abnormal slow wave activity in the human brain. *J Neurosci Methods* 2007; **163**: 119–127.
67. Fehr T, Kissler J, Moratti S, Wienbruch C, Rockstroh B, Elbert T. Source distribution of neuromagnetic slow waves and MEG-delta activity in schizophrenic patients. *Biol Psychiatry* 2001; **50**: 108–116.
68. Fehr T, Kissler J, Wienbruch C, *et al.* Source distribution of neuromagnetic slow-wave activity in schizophrenic patients – effects of activation. *Schizophr Res* 2003; **63**: 63–71.
69. Wienbruch C, Moratti S, Elbert T, *et al.* Source distribution of neuromagnetic slow wave activity in schizophrenic and depressive patients. *Clin Neurophysiol* 2003; **114**: 2052–2060.
70. Rockstroh BS, Wienbruch C, Ray WJ, Elbert T. Abnormal oscillatory brain dynamics in schizophrenia: a sign of deviant communication in neural network? *BMC Psychiatry* 2007; **7**: 44.
71. Crow TJ. Temporal lobe asymmetries as the key to the etiology of schizophrenia. *Schizophr Bull* 1990; **16**: 433–443.
72. Crow TJ. Handedness, language lateralisation and anatomical asymmetry: relevance of protocadherin XY to hominid speciation and the aetiology of psychosis. Point of view. *Br J Psychiatry* 2002; **181**: 295–297.
73. Reite M, Teale P, Goldstein L, Whalen J, Linnville S. Late auditory magnetic sources may differ in the left hemisphere of schizophrenic patients. A preliminary report. *Arch Gen Psychiatry* 1989; **46**: 565–572.
74. Reite M, Sheeder J, Teale P, et al. Magnetic source imaging evidence of sex differences in cerebral lateralization in schizophrenia. *Arch Gen Psychiatry* 1997; **54**: 433–440.
75. Rojas DC, Bawn SD, Carlson JP, Arciniegas DB, Teale PD, Reite ML. Alterations in tonotopy and auditory cerebral asymmetry in schizophrenia. *Biol Psychiatry* 2002; **52**: 32–39.
76. Teale P, Carlson J, Rojas D, Reite M. Reduced laterality of the source locations for generators of the auditory steady-state field in schizophrenia. *Biol Psychiatry* 2003; **54**: 1149–1153.
77. Rojas DC, Slason E, Teale PD, Reite ML. Neuromagnetic evidence of broader auditory cortical tuning in schizophrenia. *Schizophr Res* 2007; **97**: 206–214.
78. Reite M, Teale P, Rojas DC, Sheeder J, Arciniegas D. Schizoaffective disorder: evidence for reversed cerebral asymmetry. *Biol Psychiatry* 1999; **46**: 133–136.
79. Reite M, Teale P, Rojas DC, Benkers TL, Carlson J. Anomalous somatosensory cortical localization in schizophrenia. *Am J Psychiatry* 2003; **160**: 2148–2153.
80. Goldstein JM, Seidman LJ, O'Brien LM, *et al.* Impact of normal sexual dimorphisms on sex differences in structural brain abnormalities in schizophrenia assessed by magnetic resonance imaging. *Arch Gen Psychiatry* 2002; **59**: 154–164.

81. Hajek M, Huonker R, Boehle C, Volz HP, Nowak H, Sauer H. Abnormalities of auditory evoked magnetic fields and structural changes in the left hemisphere of male schizophrenics – a magnetoencephalographic-magnetic resonance imaging study. *Biol Psychiatry* 1997; **42**: 609–616.

82. Rockstroh B, Clementz BA, Pantev C, Blumenfeld LD, Sterr A, Elbert T. Failure of dominant left-hemispheric activation to right-ear stimulation in schizophrenia. *Neuroreport* 1998; **9**: 3819–3822.

83. Tiihonen J, Katila H, Pekkonen E, *et al.* Reversal of cerebral asymmetry in schizophrenia measured with magnetoencephalography. *Schizophr Res* 1998; **30**: 209–219.

84. Fernandez A, Rodriguez-Palancas A, Lopez-Ibor M, *et al.* Increased occipital delta dipole density in major depressive disorder determined by magnetoencephalo-graphy. *J Psychiatry Neurosci* 2005; **30**: 17–23.

85. Moratti S, Rubio G, Campo P, Keil A, Ortiz T. Hypofunction of right temporopa-rietal cortex during emotional arousal in depression. *Arch Gen Psych* 2008; **65**: 532–541.

86. Amo C, Quesney LF, Ortiz T, *et al.* Limbic paroxysmal magnetoencephalographic activity in 12 obsessive-compulsive disorder patients: a new diagnostic finding. *J Clin Psychiatry* 2004; **65**: 156–162.

87. Maihöfner C, Sperling W, Kaltenhauser M, *et al.* Spontaneous magnetoencephalo-graphic activity in patients with obsessive-compulsive disorder. *Brain Res* 2007; **1129**: 200–205.

88. Ray WJ, Odenwald M, Neuner F, *et al.* Decoupling neural networks from reality: dissociative experiences in torture victims are reflected in abnormal brain waves in left frontal cortex. *Psychol Sci.* 2006; **17**: 825–829.

89. Kolassa IT, Wienbruch C, Neuner F, *et al.* Altered oscillatory brain dynamics after repeated traumatic stress. *BMC Psychiatry* 2007; **17**: 56.

90. Hoke M, Feldmann H, Pantev C, Lutkenhoner B, Lehnertz K. Objective evidence of tinnitus in auditory evoked magnetic fields. *Hear Res* 1989; **37**: 281–286.

91. Jacobson GP, Ahmad BK, Moran J, Newman CW, Tepley N, Wharton J. Auditory evoked cortical magnetic field (M100-M200) measurements in tinnitus and normal groups. *Hear Res* 1991; **56**: 44–52.

92. Colding-Jorgensen E, Lauritzen M, Johnsen NJ, Mikkelsen KB, Saermark K. On the evidence of auditory evoked magnetic fields as an objective measure of tinnitus. *Electroencephalogr Clin Neurophysiol* 1992; **83**: 322–327.

93. Emmerich E, Richter F, Hagner H, Giessler F, Gehrlein S, Dieroff HG. Effects of discotheque music on audiometric results and central acoustic evoked neuromag-netic responses. *Int Tinnitus J* 2002; **8**: 13–19.

94. Muhlnickel W, Elbert T, Taub E, Flor H. Reorganization of auditory cortex in tinnitus. *Proc Natl Acad Sci USA* 1998; **95**: 10340–10343.

95. Wienbruch C, Paul I, Weisz N, Elbert T, Roberts LE. Frequency organization of the 40-Hz auditory steady-state response in normal hearing and in tinnitus. *NeuroImage* 2006; **33**: 180–194.

96. Weisz N, Wienbruch C, Dohrmann K, Elbert T. Neuromagnetic indicators of auditory cortical reorganization of tinnitus. *Brain* 2005; **128**: 2722–2731.

97. Weisz N, Muller S, Schlee W, Dohrmann K, Hartmann T, Elbert T. The neural code of auditory phantom perception. *J Neurosci* 2007; **27**: 1479–1484.

98. Bowyer SM, Seidman MD, Moran JE, *et al*. Coherence analysis of brain activity associated with tinnitus. In: *Biomag 2008. Proceedings of the 16th International Conference on Biomagnetism*; 2008 August, Sendai, Japan.

99. Timmermann L, Gross J, Dirks M, Volkmann J, Freund HJ, Schnitzler A. The cerebral oscillatory network of parkinsonian resting tremor. *Brain* 2003; **126**: 199–212.

100. Timmermann L, Gross J, Butz M, Kircheis G, Haussinger D, Schnitzler A. Pathological oscillatory coupling within the human motor system in different tremor syndromes as revealed by magnetoencephalography. *Neurol Clin Neurophysiol* 2004; **2004**: 26.

101. Cover KS, Vrenken H, Geurts JJ, *et al*. Multiple sclerosis patients show a highly significant decrease in alpha band interhemispheric synchronization measured using MEG. *NeuroImage* 2006; **29**: 783–788.

102. Kotini A, Anninos P, Tamiolakis D. MEG mapping in multiple sclerosis patients. *Eura Medicophys* 2007; **43**: 345–348.

103. Georgopoulos AP, Karageorgiou E, Leuthold AC, *et al*. Synchronous neural interactions assessed by magnetoencephalography: a functional biomarker for brain disorders. *J Neural Eng* 2007; **4**: 349–355.

104. de Jongh A, de Munck JC, Baayen JC, Jonkman EJ, Heethaar RM, van Dijk BW. The localization of spontaneous brain activity: first results in patients with cerebral tumors. *Clin Neurophysiol* 2001; **112**: 378–385.

105. Kamada K, Moller M, Saguer M, *et al*. A combined study of tumor-related brain lesions using MEG and proton MR spectroscopic imaging. *J Neurol Sci* 2001; **186**: 13–21.

106. Baayen JC, de Jongh A, Stam CJ, *et al*. Localization of slow wave activity in patients with tumor-associated epilepsy. *Brain Topogr* 2003; **16**: 85–93.

107. Oshino S, Kato A, Wakayama A, Taniguchi M, Hirata M, Yoshimine T. Magnetoencephalographic analysis of cortical oscillatory activity in patients with brain tumors: synthetic aperture magnetometry (SAM) functional imaging of delta band activity. *NeuroImage* 2007; **34**: 957–964.

108. de Jongh A, Baayen JC, de Munck JC, Heethaar RM, Vandertop WP, Stam CJ. The influence of brain tumor treatment on pathological delta activity in MEG. *NeuroImage* 2003; **20**: 2291–2301.

109. Stippich C, Kassubek J, Kober H, Soros P, Vieth JB. Time course of focal slow wave activity in transient ischemic attacks and transient global amnesia as measured by magnetoencephalography. *Neuroreport* 2000; **11**: 3309–3313.

110. Tecchio F, Zappasodi F, Pasqualetti P, *et al*. Rhythmic brain activity at rest from rolandic areas in acute mono-hemispheric stroke: a magnetoencephalographic study. *NeuroImage* 2005; **28**: 72–83.

111. Seki S, Nakasato N, Ohtomo S, Kanno A, Shimizu H, Tominaga T. Neuromagnetic measurement of unilateral temporo-parietal theta rhythm in patients with internal carotid artery occlusive disease. *NeuroImage* 2005; **25**: 502–510.

112. Tecchio F, Zappasodi F, Tombini M, *et al*. Brain plasticity in recovery from stroke: an MEG assessment. *NeuroImage* 2006; **32**: 1326–1334.

113. Castillo EM, Butler IJ, Baumgartner JE, Passaro A, Papanicolaou AC. When epilepsy interferes with word comprehension: findings in Landau–Kleffner syndrome. *J Child Neurol* 2008; **23**: 97–101.

114. Rossini PM, Tecchio F, Pizzella V, Lupoi D, Cassetta E, Pasqualetti P. Interhemispheric differences of sensory hand areas after monohemispheric stroke: MEG/MRI integrative study. *NeuroImage* 2001; **14**: 474–485.

115. Tecchio F, Zappasodi F, Tombini M, Caulo M, Vernieri F, Rossini PM. Interhemispheric asymmetry of primary hand representation and recovery after stroke: a MEG study. *NeuroImage* 2007; **36**: 1057–1064.

116. Breier JI, Castillo EM, Boake C, *et al.* Spatiotemporal patterns of language-specific brain activity in patients with chronic aphasia after stroke using magnetoencephalography. *NeuroImage* 2004; **23**: 1308–1316.

117. Breier JI, Billingsley-Marshall R, Pataraia E, Castillo EM, Papanicolaou AC. Magnetoencephalographic studies of language reorganization after cerebral insult. *Arch Phys Med Rehabil* 2006; **87**: S77–S83.

118. Meinzer M, Elbert T, Wienbruch C, Djundja D, Barthel G, Rockstroh B. Intensive language training enhances brain plasticity in chronic aphasia. *BMC Biol* 2004; **2**: 20.

Index